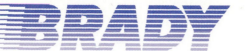

Advanced Life Support Skills

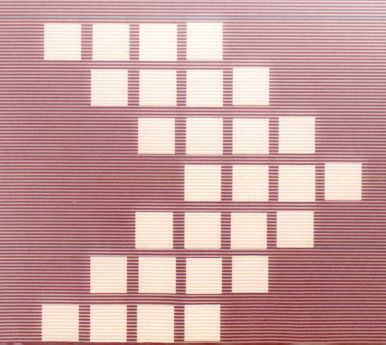

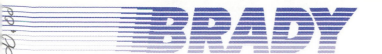

Advanced Life Support Skills

Heather Davis, MS, NREMT-P

Baxter Larmon, PhD, MICP

Scott R. Snyder, BS, NREMT-P
Contributing Editor

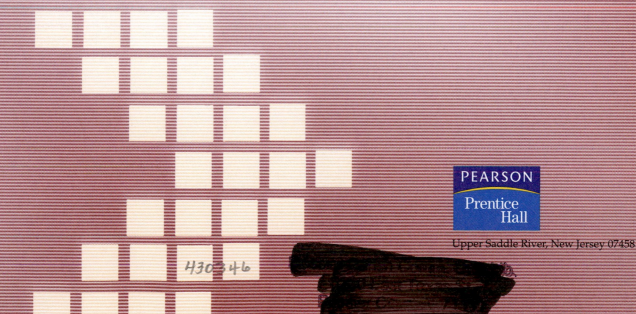

PEARSON
Prentice Hall

Upper Saddle River, New Jersey 07458

430346

Library of Congress Cataloging-in-Publication Data
Davis, Heather.
Advanced life support skills / Heather Davis, Baxter Larmon.
p. ; cm.
Includes index.
ISBN 0-13-093874-2
1.   Emergency medicine. 2.   Emergency medical technicians. 3.   Life support systems (Critical
care) I.   Davis, Heather. II.   Title.
[DNLM: 1.   Emergency Treatment—methods. 2.   Emergency Medical Technicians. 3.
Resuscitation—methods. WB 105 L324a 2007]
RC86.7.L37 2007
616.02′5—dc22
2006011995

Publisher: Julie Levin Alexander
Publisher's Assistant: Regina Bruno
Executive Editor: Marlene McHugh Pratt
Senior Managing Editor for Development: Lois Berlowitz
Assistant Editor: Matthew Sirinides
Project Development: Triple SSS Press Media Development, Inc.
Director of Marketing: Karen Allman
Executive Marketing Manager: Katrin Beacom
Marketing Coordinator: Michael Sirinides
Managing Editor for Production: Patrick Walsh
Production Liaison: Faye Gemmellaro
Production Editor: Lindsey Hancock/Carlisle Publishing Services
Manufacturing Manager: Ilene Sanford
Manufacturing Buyer: Pat Brown
Senior Design Coordinator: Christopher Weigand
Cover Design: Christopher Weigand
Cover Photo: Getty Images
Interior Design: Mary Siener
Composition: Carlisle Publishing Services
Printing and Binding: Banta/Menasha
Cover Printer: Coral Graphics

Studentaid.ed.gov, the U.S. Department of Education's Website on college planning assistance, is a valuable tool for anyone intending to pursue higher education. Designed to help students at all stages of schooling, including international students, returning students, and parents, it is a guide to the financial aid process. This Website presents information on applying to and attending college, as well as on funding your education and repaying loans. It also provides links to useful resources, such as state education agency contact information, assistance in filling out financial aid forms, and an introduction to various forms of student aid.

NOTICE ON CARE PROCEDURES
This text reflects current EMS practices based on the 1998 U.S. Department of Transportation's EMT-Paramedic National Standard Curriculum. It is the intent of the authors and publisher that this manual be used as part of a formal Emergency Medical Technician-Paramedic education program taught by qualified instructors and supervised by a licensed physician. The procedures described in this manual are based upon consultation with EMS and medical authorities. The authors and publisher have taken care to make certain that these procedures reflect currently accepted clinical practice; however, they cannot be considered absolute recommendations. The material in this manual contains the most current information available at the time of publication. However, federal, state, and local guidelines concerning clinical practices, including, without limitation, those governing infection control and universal precautions, change rapidly. The reader should note, therefore, that the new regulations may require changes in some procedures. It is the responsibility of the reader to familiarize himself or herself with the policies and procedures set by federal, state, and local agencies as well as the institution or agency where the reader is employed. The authors and the publisher of this manual disclaim any liability, loss, or risk resulting directly or indirectly from the suggested procedures and theory, from any undetected errors, or from the reader's misunderstanding of the text. It is the reader's responsibility to stay informed of any new changes or recommendations made by any federal, state, and local agency as well as by his or her employing institution or agency.

Pearson Education Ltd.
Pearson Education Singapore, Pte. Ltd.
Pearson Education Canada, Ltd.
Pearson Education—Japan

Pearson Education Australia PTY, Limited
Pearson Education North Asia Ltd.
Pearson Educación de Mexico, S.A. de C.V.
Pearson Education Malaysia, Pte. Ltd.
Pearson Education, Upper Saddle River, New Jersey

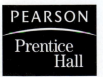

10 9 8 7 6 5 4 3 2 1
ISBN 0-13-093874-2

DEDICATION

"To Ricky, for knowing that encouragement is like oxygen to the soul."
—Heather Davis

"In loving memory of my parents. To all my past, present, and future students."
—Baxter Larmon

Contents

THE AUTHORS

Heather Davis, MS, NREMT-P

Heather Davis is the Education Program Director for the Los Angeles County Fire Department, where she manages the primary EMT and continuing education programs for over 3,000 EMTs and paramedics. Her previous position was as the Clinical Coordinator for the UCLA Center for Prehospital Care, where she continues to lecture and be active in primary paramedic education. Ms. Davis has been involved in patient care and education activities in rural Iowa, suburban New York, and the Rocky Mountains of Colorado. She has worked in disaster response, critical incident management, and tactical EMS. Ms. Davis served on the Board of Directors for National Association of EMS Educators (NAEMSE) and is the Prehospital Trauma Life Support State Coordinator for California. She holds a Master of Science degree from New York Medical College and is a published author and national speaker.

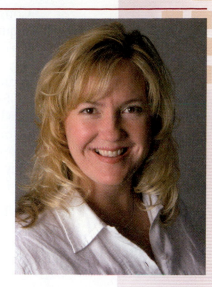

Baxter Larmon, PhD, MICP

Dr. Baxter Larmon is a Professor of Medicine at the University of California at Los Angeles (UCLA) School of Medicine and is the Director of the UCLA Center for Prehospital Care. He has more than 30 years of experience with emergency medical services. He is the founding director of the Prehospital Care Research Forum and served on the founding Board of Directors of the National Association of EMS Educators (NAEMSE). Dr. Larmon is both nationally and internationally recognized as an EMS educator. He has spoken at more than 500 EMS conferences and has written more than 70 publications in emergency medicine.

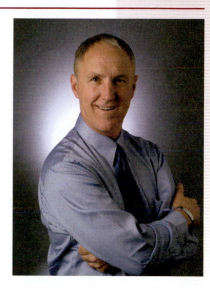

PREFACE

Congratulations! By purchasing this book you have demonstrated a commitment to acquiring the technical expertise associated with being an ALS provider. The actual job of providing emergency prehospital care is complex and dynamic. However, gaining and maintaining excellence in the fundamental skills of the job will improve your confidence and competence as you provide care to patients in emergency situations.

Intended as a resource for skills and procedures common to the practice of EMS, this book covers advanced life support (ALS) skills. There are hundreds of photos illustrating the proper procedural steps for each skill. A CD package is also available to support this book. The CDs actually demonstrate each skill in real time, which you may find helpful in learning and practicing the ALS procedures.

Each skill has several features that will enhance your use of this book.

▶ The *assessment* and *ongoing assessment* precede and follow each *step-by-step procedure* and will assist you in gathering pertinent information from the patient prior to and after engaging in the skill. In most cases, the assessment actually helps you determine whether or not that particular skill is indicated for your patient. The ongoing assessment helps you with the proper follow-up to make sure that the procedure has been a success.

▶ The *rationale* imbedded into the procedural steps helps you understand why each step is to be done the way it is described, or why it is important.

▶ Also, pay particular attention to the *problem solving* section. For every procedure there exist possible complications or pitfalls to correctly completing the skill. The problem solving section should help you develop alternative approaches when problems arise.

▶ *Pediatric and geriatric notes* highlight particular issues and potential pitfalls with these populations.

▶ Finally, each chapter has a *case study* to help you tie it all together.

These skills are presented using the most generic or broad-based equipment possible. When an EMS system chooses a particular piece of equipment, you should follow the manufacturer's recommendations for use to ensure your safety and the safety of your patient. In some cases, specific manufacturer instructions could alter the steps presented here. Your instructor or training officer is a good resource whenever a discrepancy arises. He or she should be familiar with national standards, state or local protocol, or the procedure set forth by your medical director.

ACKNOWLEDGMENTS

We wish to acknowledge the efforts of the following individuals who reviewed the *Advanced Life Support Skills* manuscript.

Reviewers

John L. Beckman, AA, FF/PM Instructor
Addision Fire Protection District
EMS Instructor at Technical Center of DuPage County
Addison, IL

Diana Cave, RN, MSN
Portland Community College
Institute for Health Professionals
AHA Community Training Center Director
Portland, Oregon

Tony Crystal, ScD, EMT-P, RPhT
Director, Emergency Medical Services
Lake Land College
Mattoon, IL

Dr. Grant Goold
American River College
Citrus Heights, CA

Raymond Klein
EMS Training Director
Public Safety and Emergency Services Institute
Pima Community College
Tucson, AZ

Darren P. Lacroix
Del Mar College
Corpus Christi, TX

James S. Lion, Jr., EMT
Emergency Medical Services for the State of New York
EMT Instructor
Williamsville, NY

Brittany Martinelli
Santa Fe Community College
Gainesville, FL

Justin McCullough, BS, EMT-P
Clinical Skills Coordinator UCLA-DFH Paramedic Education

Steve Myers, RN, CEN, EMT-P
EMS Department Chair
Indian River Community College
Ft. Pierce, FL

Norma Pancake
EMS Coordinator
Pierce County EMS Office
Pierce County Emergency Management
Tacoma, WA

Brian J. Wilson, BA, EMT-P
Education Director
Texas Tech University, Health Sciences Center at El Paso
El Paso, TX

Contributor

Our appreciation to Scott R. Snyder BS, NREMT-P, for his substantial contributions to both the photo preparation and to the text material.

Photo Shoot Coordination

We would also like to thank the following people for their outstanding help on this project: Marc Burdick (Santa Barbara County EMS Agency), Richard Battle (Los Angeles County Fire Dept.), Eileen Ehinger (Keystone Medical Center), Madeline Ridenhour, Braden Burr, and Gabriel Wilner.

Thank you to these special people from Summit County Ambulance Service, Summit County, Colorado, who allowed Brady to use their facilities and who modeled for us: Laura Mignone, Kim Campbell, Edward Parry, George Rohwer, Phil McFall, Patricia Fanning, and Jennifer Calhoun.

Thank you to the following people from Lake Dillion Fire-Rescue who lent their services: Chris Nelson, Patrick Grout, Joseph Delmore, and Jack Strong.

ADVANCED AIRWAY MANAGEMENT SKILLS

Few would disagree that airway management is one of the most important, and arguably the only truly life-*saving*, skills emergency medical service (EMS) providers have. Although this section focuses on advanced airway procedures, good basic life support (BLS) skills in airway management are paramount, and should always be performed *first*, before advanced life support (ALS) management techniques are employed. You will find that often no ALS procedures are needed if the provider's BLS techniques are well practiced and executed accurately in the patient's time of need.

However, circumstances do exist when BLS attempts to manage the airway are not sufficient. Endotracheal intubation is still the gold standard for securing the patient's airway. Placing a tube in the trachea not only allows you to ventilate and oxygenate the patient's lungs, but allows you to protect the patient from aspirating stomach contents, which can be deadly. Sometimes an airway obstruction caused by choking or trauma may prevent placement of an endotracheal tube, in which case the paramedic can perform a needle cricothyroidotomy, another life-saving intervention. Similarly, a tension pneumothorax will quickly impede both respiratory and cardiac functions unless the pressure is released with a needle decompression of the chest. This section will walk you through each of the previously mentioned procedures and many more as you learn advanced techniques in airway management.

CHAPTER 1

Endotracheal Intubation

KEY TERMS

Bag-valve mask

Carina

Cricoid pressure

Cuffed endotracheal tubes

Hypercapnic

Hyperventilate

Hypoxemic

Hypoxia

Lumen

Macintosh blade

Magill forceps

Miller blade

Nasopharyngeal

Oropharyngeal airway

Patent

Pneumothorax

Preoxygenate

Sellick's maneuver

Stylette

Uncuffed endotracheal
tubes

Vallecula

OBJECTIVES

The student will be able to do the following:

▶ List the indications for performing endotracheal intubation (pp. 1–8).

▶ Describe the importance of properly performing endotracheal intubation (pp. 1–8).

▶ Describe the proper technique for performing endotracheal intubation (pp. 9–12).

▶ Demonstrate the ability to properly perform endotracheal intubation (pp. 9–12).

INTRODUCTION

Endotracheal intubation (ETI), the inserting of an endotracheal tube (ETT) into the trachea, is unparalleled in its ability to secure and control a compromised airway, earning it the reputation as the "gold standard" of airway maintenance. Intubation is a skill that requires knowledge, ability, and hours of practice before proficiency is obtained. In addition, continuing education, regular practice, and performance review throughout one's career is essential to prevent the deterioration of this valuable skill. Patient's lives will depend on your ability to secure and control the compromised airway.

Intubation can be performed in several ways, with some of the more common methods including the oral, nasal, or surgical routes. In this ability review, we will discuss and illustrate orotracheal intubation. There are several indications for intubation, including respiratory or cardiac arrest, respiratory distress secondary to trauma or disease, unconsciousness or altered mental status resulting in an absent gag reflex, and impending airway occlusion secondary to airway burns, anaphylaxis, or foreign body obstruction.

Contraindications to intubation include the presence of a permanent tracheostomy, or any situation where attempts at intubation could induce laryngospasm. In addition, the presence of a gag reflex is a contraindication to orotracheal intubation, and an indication for nasotracheal or rapid sequence intubation (RSI).

Along with the indications and contraindications, you should be familiar with the complications of ETI, which include **hypoxia** due to prolonged intubation attempts, esophageal intubation, and mainstem bronchus intubation. Right mainstem bronchus intubation is more common due to its larger diameter and more continuous path with the trachea, compared to the left. Other complications associated with ETI are laryngospasm, aspiration, vagal stimulation causing arrhythmia, injury to the upper airway structures due to aggressive intubation techniques and then, finally, trauma to the vocal cords and broken teeth.

The advantages of endotracheal intubation are significant. Not only does ETI isolate the trachea, permitting complete control of the airway, but it also removes the esophagus as a possible conduit for air movement, eliminating gastric insufflation and distension, as well as decreasing the possibility of passive regurgitation. ETI also eliminates the difficult procedure of holding a mask seal, requiring one less provider for optimal airway maintenance.

In addition, the ETT serves as a medication administration route, allowing for the administration of oxygen, lidocaine, epinephrine, atropine, and narcan (OLEAN). Some sources also recognize diazepam as a medication that can be administered via the ETT, but this remains controversial. Vasopressin is another advanced life support drug that can be administered down the ETT, though, again, absorption of any medication down the ETT is not as reliable as through other routes, such as intravenous (IV) and IO access.

There are several pieces of equipment needed to perform intubation, which should be checked and readied prior to your intubation attempt. First you need to make sure that you have proper body substance isolation (BSI) equipment, including gloves, goggles, and a face mask or face shield. Some providers even choose to don a gown, time permitting, to prevent contamination of their uniform.

Prior to checking and preparing the equipment needed for endotracheal intubation, you should prepare your patient. Ensure that the patient has a **patent** BLS airway and is either ventilating adequately on his own and receiving 100 percent oxygen via a nonrebreather mask, is being assisted with a **bag-valve mask** (BVM) and 100 percent oxygen if ventilation is inadequate, or is being provided positive-pressure ventilation with 100 percent oxygen in cases of apnea.

Proper positioning of the patient's airway includes the head tilt-chin lift used in concert with head elevation to open the airway and assist in the visualization of the vocal cords during intubation (Figure 1.1). Padding may be required beneath the patient's head and neck in order to create the proper axis for intubation. Head elevation is accomplished by placing pillows, towels, or blankets under the head to support a position that places the patient's ear canal at the level of the sternal notch, when viewed from the lateral perspective (Figure 1.2). This position is often referred to as the "sniffing" position, and aligns the oral, pharyngeal, and tracheal axis allowing for better visualization of the glottis. Obviously, this positioning is contraindicated in patients with suspected cervical spine injuries.

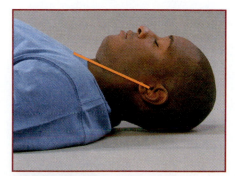

Figure 1.1

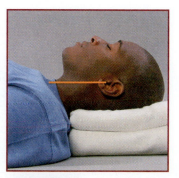

Figure 1.2

Use of an **oropharyngeal airway** (OPA) is recommended in those patients who appear to be unconscious, as it is a great therapeutic as well as diagnostic tool; therapeutic because it removes the tongue as an airway obstruction, and diagnostic because it gives you information on the patient's ability to protect his airway. If a patient accepts an OPA without gagging, he cannot protect the airway and most likely will require ETI sometime in the immediate future if his condition does not rapidly improve.

It is not necessary to **hyperventilate** a patient during the entire pre-intubation period unless the patient has sustained a closed-head injury and you suspect increased intracranial pressure. Rather, your goal should be to **preoxygenate** your patient prior to your ETI attempt. This is best accomplished by ventilating your patient with a tidal volume sufficient to produce normal chest rise and fall, at a rate of 8-10 times per minute, taking about one second per ventilation using the BVM.

Applying **cricoid pressure,** also known as **Sellick's maneuver,** during BVM ventilation can help reduce the incidence of gastric insufflation and passive regurgitation of stomach contents. In addition, it may or may not allow for a better view of the larynx during the intubation attempt. The use of a pulse oximeter can help with assessing the success of preoxygenation in patients with a pulse, and the individuals providing BLS airway control should attempt to achieve a SaO_2 as close to 100 percent as possible. In patients without a pulse, evaluation of chest rise and fall, mask seal, BVM compliance, and skin color will be a better indication of the effectiveness of ventilations.

Proper BLS airway control should be considered an integral part of the preparation for ETI. Ensure the patient is well oxygenated before you begin your intubation attempt. Do not allow the patient to desaturate. If you notice the pulse oximeter reading falling, suspend your intubation attempt and ventilate the patient.

You will need to prepare your intubation tool, the laryngoscope, which consists of a handle and a blade. The handle houses the batteries that power the light source in the laryngoscope. In older laryngoscope models, the light bulb is attached to the end of the laryngoscope blade. When the blade is secured to the handle (Figure 1.3) and elevated to a 90° angle, the electrical connection is completed and the light goes on (Figure 1.4). When checking your laryngoscope, you want to make sure that the blade attaches firmly to the handle and that the light is tight (bulb is firmly attached), white (not yellow with age or use), and bright (not dim or wavering in intensity, indicating low battery power). This is very important because you are about to go into a place where it is dark, and you do not want the light bulb falling off into the patient's throat or the light going out while you are trying to intubate.

After checking the light, collapse the blade against the handle to turn off the light (Figure 1.5), leave it attached, and set it aside in a safe area. In the newer, fiber-optic laryngoscopes, a light bulb is located in the laryngoscope handle, and light travels

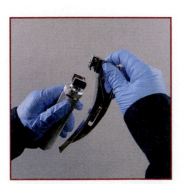

Figure 1.3

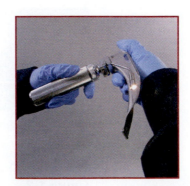

Figure 1.4

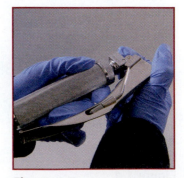

Figure 1.5

through a fiber-optic channel to the distal end of the blade. Handles and blades may be reusable with proper cleaning after use, or may be disposable.

There are many different types of laryngoscope blades, but the two most commonly used in the prehospital environment are the **Macintosh** (curved) **blade** and the **Miller** (straight) **blade** (Figure 1.6). Both range in size from 0 for infants through 4 for large adults.

The Macintosh blade is designed to be inserted into the hypopharynx, with the tip placed into the **vallecula** (Figure 1.7). Insertion of the tip into the vallecula and applying pressure to the hypoepiglottic ligament results in lifting of the epiglottis and better visualization of the glottic opening. The curved shape and wide flange of the Macintosh blade allows for better tongue control when compared to the Miller blade.

The Miller blade is designed to be placed in the hypopharynx and its distal tip used to directly lift the epiglottis (Figure 1.8), allowing for an unobstructed view of the glottic opening. The Miller blade is often used in trauma patients, or any other patient who cannot be placed in the "sniffing position," as its straight shape allows for an extra half centimeter or so of lift (Figure 1.9), which may prove to be the difference between seeing the glottic opening or not. Many users also prefer the Miller blade over the Macintosh blade for pediatric patients, as it affords greater control of the large, floppy epiglottis typical of this population. Ultimately, with practice and experience using both blades, you will acquire a preference based on your particular technique, but you should become familiar with whichever laryngoscope blades are made available for your use.

Once you have checked your laryngoscope, make sure that a suction unit is ready and on, you have the appropriate suction catheter for the situation, and you have a set of **Magill forceps** readily available should you need them. Magill forceps (Figure 1.10) are used to remove a foreign body airway obstruction (FBAO)

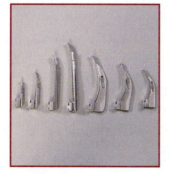

Figure 1.6

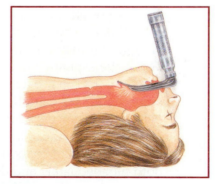

Figure 1.7

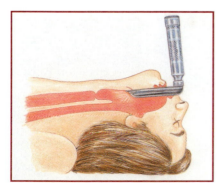

Figure 1.8

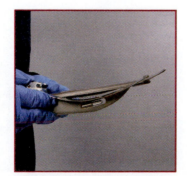

Figure 1.9

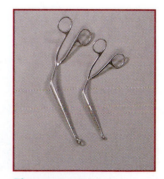

Figure 1.10

from the airway should one be identified. The Magill forceps are a specially shaped pair of clamps with a long neck and circular tips with serrated inner surfaces. They are designed to be used in the oro- and laryngopharynx along with the laryngoscope blade to retrieve foreign objects. They also come in a small size for pediatric patients and a larger size for adults.

Finally, you will need to pick an appropriately sized ET tube and prepare it for intubation. ET tubes come in several sizes ranging from 2.5 for neonates to 9.0 for larger adults (Figure 1.11). It is important to pick the correct size tube so as not to damage the patient's airway. In an adult, the narrowest portion of the upper airway is at the vocal cords or glottic opening. These limitations are what determine what size diameter or lumen tube to use. This can be determined by the law of averages for sizes. A female adult is usually around the 6.5–7.5 size ETT, and the male adult is usually a 7.0–8.0 size ETT. The numbers indicate the **lumen** size, or inner diameter, of the tube itself, measured in millimeters.

Another way to size the tube is by taking the pinky finger of the patient, and making sure that it is the same as the outer diameter or lumen of the ETT. Do not use your own pinky, because it may be smaller or bigger than the patient's. This helps to ensure that the tube will be able to go past the vocal cords when trying to place the ETT. If resistance is met because the tube diameter is too big, then do not force the issue, or the tube; just get a smaller size ETT. The lengths of the tubes range from 12 cm to 32 cm. When intubating, it is not necessary to place the entire length of the tube down the trachea, but rather simply place the cuff 1–2 cm past the vocal cords. Some ET tubes will have an indicator as to where the level of the vocal cords should correlate on the tube, helping to prevent passing the ETT too far, resulting in intubation of the mainstem bronchi. All ETTs will have a ruler, graduated in centimeters, along the length to aid in identifying tube insertion depth, often recorded at the patient's incisor teeth. The distal end of the ETT is beveled to help prevent occlusion, and a "Murphy's eye," or hole (Figure 1.12), is located about 1 cm proximal to the ETT tip as a failsafe, should the distal end become occluded.

Some **endotracheal tubes** are **uncuffed** (typically those size 5.5 and smaller), and others are **cuffed** (typically those 6.0 and larger). The cuff is an inflatable balloon at the distal end of the tube that helps to seal off the trachea, preventing any air leakage or the aspiration of secretions or vomitus. While the cuff is helpful in anchoring down the ETT in the trachea after a successful intubation, the tube should always be secured in place using some type of after market device or tape to maintain proper placement. The cuff holds approximately 10 cc of air, and is inflated by attaching a 10-cc syringe to the inflation valve located proximal on the pilot balloon (Figure 1.13). The cuff and pilot balloon should be checked prior to intubation to ensure that they both fill adequately and do not leak. It is common practice to leave the ETT in and squeeze the cuff through the packaging to avoid contamination.

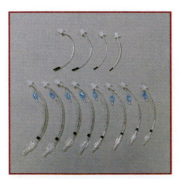

Figure 1.11

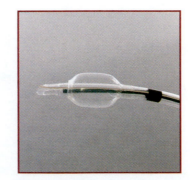

Figure 1.12

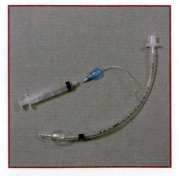

Figure 1.13

A **stylette** is a malleable plastic-covered metal wire that is inserted into the ETT to provide greater control of the distal end of the ETT (Figure 1.14). The stylette also allows for shaping of the ETT to aid in intubation. There are many variations of tube shapes that can be utilized, but recent evidence suggests that a "straight to cuff," or "hockey stick" shape, results in higher intubation success rates as it does not obstruct your view of the glottic opening than does the traditional "curved" shape (Figure 1.15). The stylette should be inserted into the ETT to a depth about 2 cm above the tip of the tube, above the Murphy's eye, in order to prevent it from projecting from the distal ETT and causing injury. The photo displays an improper placement (Figure 1.16).

To summarize the equipment preparation for ETI:

▶ Ensure that proper BLS airway maintenance and ventilation with 100 percent oxygen is provided, cricoid pressure is being applied, and that a pulse oximeter is being utilized.

▶ Select a proper-sized laryngoscope blade for your particular patient, ensure that it fits securely on the laryngoscope handle, and verify the light is white, bright, and tight.

▶ Select an endotracheal tube of the proper size for your patient, and with the tube in the wrapping material attach a 10-cc syringe to the pilot balloon, inflate the balloon and the cuff with approximately 10 cc of air, ensure that there are no leaks, then deflate the balloon, leaving the syringe attached and the tube in the wrapper to prevent contamination.

▶ Insert a stylette to a depth about 2 cm proximal to the distal end of the ETT, then bend the ETT to a "straight to cuff" shape.

▶ Ensure that you have a working suction unit by your side with an appropriate suction catheter for the situation, and that your Magill forceps are nearby should you require them.

Once you and your equipment are prepared, move to the patient's head while instructing the person providing BVM ventilations to preoxygenate the patient, then move to the side, taking and holding on to the OPA, if one is being used. You can then move in and start your intubation attempt.

The potential for failure is increased exponentially when you fail to prepare for intubation. If you fail to ensure that a proper BLS airway is maintained and proper ventilations supplied, your patient will end up with gastric distension. If you forget to have a working suction unit nearby and the patient regurgitates, aspiration of vomit may occur. If you don't take the time to put a stylette in the ETT, your tube may hang up on the epiglottis and not pass through the cords. If you don't check the balloon for air leaks prior to intubation and there is one, you will have to pull a properly placed

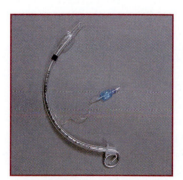

Figure 1.14

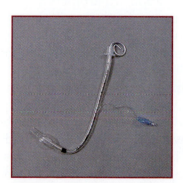

Figure 1.15

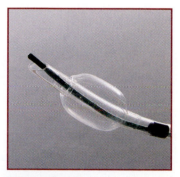

Figure 1.16

tube after the fact. Take the time to ensure that a proper BLS airway and ventilation has been established. Take the time to check and set up all of your equipment, the same way, every time. Take the time to properly prepare for intubation, every time, and give yourself the greatest likelihood of success, every time.

► EQUIPMENT

You will need the following equipment (Figure 1.17):

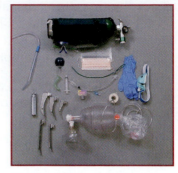

Figure 1.17

- ► Gloves
- ► Goggles
- ► Face mask
- ► Suction equipment
- ► Endotracheal tubes (various sizes)
- ► 10-cc syringe
- ► Stylette
- ► Stethoscope
- ► Bag-valve mask
- ► Laryngoscope handle (with working batteries)
- ► Laryngoscope blades (various sizes and types)
- ► Tape or commercial tube securing device
- ► Pulse oximeter
- ► Esophageal detector device
- ► Colormetric ETCO$_2$ detector or capnography

ASSESSMENT

While ETI is considered an ALS skill, the assessment of a patient requiring intubation focuses on the basics: airway, breathing, and circulation (ABCs). The most obvious assessment finding that should result in an immediate attempt to intubate is apnea secondary to respiratory or cardiac arrest. This decision can become more involved in those patients who present in severe respiratory distress or extremis secondary to disease or trauma. Signs of severe respiratory distress include increased work of breathing, accessory muscle use, decreased lung sounds and air movement, nasal flaring, cyanosis, altered mental status, decreased SaO$_2$, and alterations in ETCO$_2$ specific to the underlying disease or insult. Of course, not all patients who present with severe respiratory distress necessarily need intubation. Some patients may respond to medication administration, while others respond to noninvasive methods of breathing assistance such as continuous positive airway pressure. In addition to having severe respiratory distress, patients in extremis who are in need of ETI will be tired, bradypneic, and have a decreased level of consciousness; simply stated, these patients will be in impending respiratory arrest.

Impending airway obstruction requiring ETI can be anticipated by first recognizing that the potential exists for the development of obstruction. Patients with airway burns, anaphylaxis, or epiglottitis should be considered at high risk for the development of airway obstruction and monitored closely for the development or worsening of dysphagia, hoarse voice, stridor, and respiratory distress. As complete obstruction can develop rapidly, it is important to recognize the signs and symptoms early, have your ETI equipment prepared, and make the decision to intubate prior to total occlusion. Foreign body airway obstruction, as evidenced by apnea, cyanosis, loss of consciousness, and inability to ventilate, requires immediate foreign body removal under direct laryngoscopy.

Unconsciousness or altered mental status are not absolute indications for ETI, but are when combined with a lack of a gag reflex and a risk of aspiration. As most patients in the prehospital environment can be assumed to have some gastric content, any patient without a gag reflex you encounter is a strong candidate for ETI. Certainly, if your patient accepts an OPA and is receiving positive-pressure ventilations, ETI is indicated unless you expect rapid improvement in the patient's condition, such as a hypoglycemic patient who is about to receive dextrose or a patient with a narcotic overdose who will be administered naloxone. If these patients are vomiting and the airway is uncontrollable, however, suctioning and immediate intubation may be required.

PROCEDURE: Endotracheal Intubation

1. Take infection control precautions.

   Rationale: Gloves, goggles, and a face mask are essential equipment when working around the airway since airway secretions can transmit blood-borne pathogens.

2. Open the airway manually with either the head-tilt chin-lift technique with head elevation (Figure 1.18) or jaw thrust for trauma victims.

   Rationale: Proper positioning of the airway will assist the rescuer in eliminating the tongue as an airway obstruction, providing more adequate BVM ventilations, and visualizing the cords during endotracheal intubation.

   GERIATRIC NOTE:

   Many geriatric patients suffer from cervical disk changes, which cause their neck to be stiff and sometimes immobile. Achieving the sniffing position for these patients may be difficult and provide a challenge during intubation. Excessive force should never be used to achieve proper positioning of the head.

3. Ensure the gag reflex is absent and elevate the tongue with the insertion of an OPA (Figure 1.19).

   Rationale: When ventilating the non-intubated patient, an airway adjunct helps to eliminate the tongue as an airway obstruction. In addition, it helps assess for the presence of a gag reflex.

4. Begin ventilating the patient with a BVM attached to 100 percent oxygen at 15–25 lpm (Figure 1.20).

   Rationale: The patient is presumably **hypoxemic** and/or **hypercapnic,** and ventilation will help to correct these conditions. While room air delivers an oxygen concentration of 21 percent, high-flow,

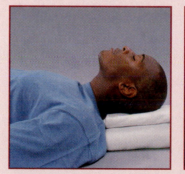 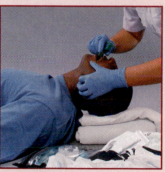

Figure 1.18   **Figure 1.19**

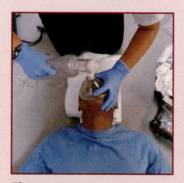

Figure 1.20

continued...

high-concentration oxygen via BVM will deliver at least 85 percent oxygen concentration, which can more quickly correct hypoxemia and hypercapnia.

5. Apply cricoid pressure, and continue ventilating. Give BVM ventilations every 5 to 6 seconds or about 10–12 breaths per minute for the perfusing patient, or 8–10 times per minute when CPR is in progress. Use enough tidal volume to achieve normal chest rise (Figure 1.21).

   Rationale: Ventilatory rates of 10–12 breaths per minute prevent blowing off too much carbon dioxide, which is dangerous because it can cause alkalosis and vasoconstriction. Ventilation volumes adequate to produce normal chest rise and fall are desirable to prevent complications such as gastric insufflation, barotrauma, and decreased venous return to the heart. Cricoid pressure helps to reduce gastric insufflation and passive regurgitation.

6. Select proper equipment for intubation to include properly sized laryngoscope blade, endotracheal tube and stylette, syringe, and tape or tube securing device (Figure 1.22).

   Rationale: Many types and sizes of equipment exist. Selecting properly sized equipment will help ensure successful tube placement.

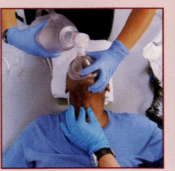

Figure 1.21

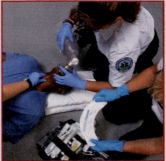

Figure 1.22

the risk of aspiration of vomit, secretions, and blood.

8. Insert a stylette into the ETT to a depth about 2 cm before the distal end, just above the Murphy's eye (Figure 1.24).

   Rationale: The stylette will provide rigidity to the ETT, and proper insertion depth is necessary to prevent injury to the airway.

9. Check the laryngoscope and light bulb by assembling the handle and blade combination to ensure the light comes on, is white and bright, and cannot be easily unscrewed from its position.

   Rationale: An improperly functioning laryngoscope will make it difficult to visualize the cords and pass the ETT.

10. Pre-oxygenate the patient for at least 30 seconds prior to the intubation attempt.

   Rationale: You will not be providing ventilation during the intubation attempt and failure to preoxygenate can worsen or cause hypoxia.

> ### GERIATRIC NOTE:
> While most adult patients can be intubated with a 7.0 or 7.5 ET tube, remember that with degenerative changes, many geriatric patients more closely resemble the size of a child. While a cuffed ET tube is still indicated, a smaller cuffed tube in the 5.5–6.5 range may provide more success.

7. Check for ET tube cuff leaks by inflating the cuff, pinching slightly to ensure no cuff tears exist, then deflating the cuff (Figure 1.23). You may leave the syringe attached to the tube at this time if you wish.

   Rationale: A patent cuff is required to provide a seal between the ETT and the trachea, reducing

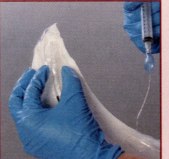

Figure 1.23

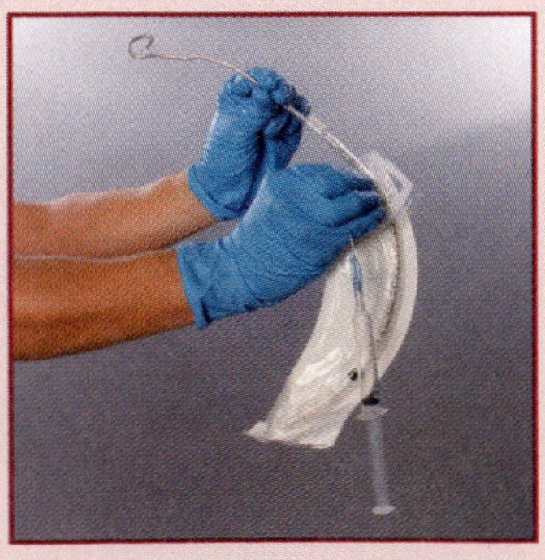

Figure 1.24

11. Remove the airway adjunct previously inserted (Figure 1.25).

    Rationale: It will be easier to visualize the cords with no obstacles in the mouth.

12. Open the patient's mouth using the "scissor" technique.

    Rationale: The scissor technique allows you to open the patient's mouth without inserting your fingers and risking a bite injury.

13. Hold the laryngoscope in your left hand, insert the laryngoscope blade on the right side of the mouth, and sweep to the left to displace the tongue (Figure 1.26).

    Rationale: Displacing the tongue to the left prevents it from obstructing your view of the vocal cords.

14. With the tip of the laryngoscope, follow the tongue into the hypopharynx, identify the epiglottis, and if using a Macintosh blade, insert the tip into the vallecula. If using a Miller blade, lift the epiglottis.

    Rationale: Each blade is designed to be used in a specific fashion.

15. Lifting upward along the axis of the laryngoscope handle and without flexing your wrist, elevate the mandible with the laryngoscope blade and visualize the vocal cords (Figure 1.27).

    Rationale: Elevating the mandible by lifting the laryngoscope allows visual access of the cords. Flexing your wrist will not elevate the mandible, but will put pressure on the teeth, potentially breaking them. If the mandible is not displaced well enough or far enough, the cords will remain obscured and no tube can be placed.

16. Introduce the ET tube while maintaining direct visualization of the vocal cords. Advance to the proper depth, which is when the tube cuff sits inferior to the vocal cords but superior to the **carina** (Figure 1.28).

    Rationale: A tube inserted too far will likely end up in the right mainstem bronchus, allowing only one lung to be inflated.

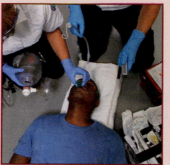
Figure 1.25

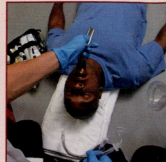
Figure 1.26

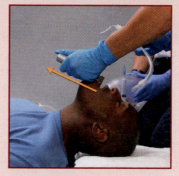
Figure 1.27

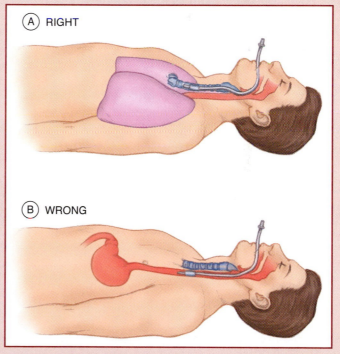

Ⓐ RIGHT

Ⓑ WRONG

Figure 1.28

continued...

17. While firmly holding the ETT at the patient's lip, remove the stylette from the ETT (Figure 1.29).

Rationale: The stylette is used only to assist in proper placement of the tube.

18. Inflate the cuff to the proper pressure (typically requiring around 10 cc), and disconnect the syringe (Figure 1.30).

Rationale: Failing to disconnect the syringe will allow air to escape from the cuff back into the syringe.

19. Direct ventilation of the patient while still manually securing the tube in place. Utilize an end-tidal carbon dioxide ($ETCO_2$) detector between the BVM and ETT to aid in confirmation of tracheal placement of the ETT (Figure 1.31).

Rationale: Use of the $ETCO_2$ detector is secondary to auscultation of lung sounds and epigastrium, but can be placed now for convenience.

20. Confirm proper tube placement by auscultating for lung sounds bilaterally over each lung (Figure 1.32) and for the absence of sounds over the epigastrium (Figure 1.33). If no lung sounds are heard, extubate the patient (see Chapter 2).

Rationale: Presence of bilateral lung sounds and absence of epigastrium sounds are a *primary indicator* of proper tube placement.

21. Use an esophageal detector device for secondary configuration of the ETT.

Rationale: Utilization of an EDD aids in recognition of misplaced or dislodged ET tubes.

22. Secure the tube in place with tape or a commercial securing device.

Rationale: Failure to secure the tube will result in tube dislodgement and a possible unrecognized esophageal intubation. Displacement of a tube into the esophagus will most likely result in the patient's death (Figure 1.34).

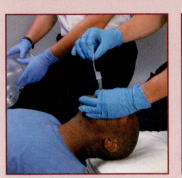
Figure 1.29

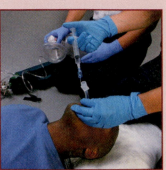
Figure 1.30

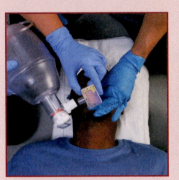
Figure 1.31

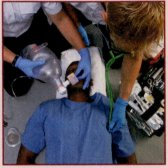
Figure 1.32

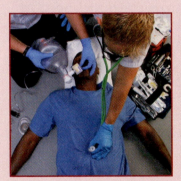
Figure 1.33

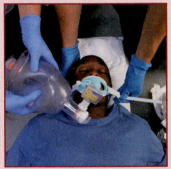
Figure 1.34

ONGOING ASSESSMENT

A patient who requires intubation is, by definition, a critical patient who requires re-assessment at least every 5 minutes. Reassessment includes not only evaluation of the vital signs and mental status, but also of the tube itself.

Lung sounds should be reassessed every time the patient is moved, and several times during transport. Any change in lung sounds or epigastric sounds can be an indication that the tube has been dislodged, and extubation may be required.

During ventilation, transport, and patient movement, it is fairly easy for the tube to accidentally be pushed further into the trachea and down into one bronchus, or pulled out and replaced into the esophagus. Noting the depth of tube insertion by using the centimeter marks on the side of the tube can help to ensure the tube is not pushed past the carina. Frequent reassessment of tube verification methods, such as chest rise, condensation in the tube, $ETCO_2$ detection, and even pulse oximetry for perfusing patients, can help to ensure the tube is still in the trachea.

▶PROBLEM SOLVING

▶ When intubating a patient with a gag reflex, use of the **nasopharyngeal** route is desirable in place of the oropharyngeal route. Orotracheal intubation in a patient with an intact gag reflex requires the used of sedative agents (facilitated intubation) or sedatives combined with paralytic agents (RSI).

▶ Be especially careful about ventilatory rates. Prehospital professionals have been proven to hyperventilate patients at rates as high as 60 times/minute, resulting in hypocapnia and increased risk of barotrauma, gastric distension, passive regurgitation, and decreased venous return.

▶ Preoxygenation before suctioning or intubation attempts is essential to prevent hypoxia. Preoxygenation takes place during the pre-intubation period and is accomplished by providing positive-pressure ventilation with 100 percent oxygen at a rate of 10-12 times per minute for perfusing patients, or 8-10 times per minute when CPR is in progress. Use enough volume to achieve normal chest rise and fall, with each ventilation taking about one second.

▶ The goal of preoxygenation is to supersaturate the blood with oxygen prior to the intubation attempt to prevent hypoxia during the intubation attempt. Monitoring pulse oximetry in patients with a pulse is useful in achieving this goal, and you should attempt to achieve a SaO_2 of 100 percent during the preoxygenation period. You should discontinue your intubation attempt and reoxygenate with positive-pressure ventilation by BVM when the patient's SaO_2 falls to 90 percent.

▶ If lung sounds are heard on only one side after intubation, the tube has likely been placed into the right or left mainstem bronchus. Try deflating the cuff and recessing the tube a few centimeters, then reinflating the tube to check for bilateral chest rise. If bilateral chest rise is still not occurring, assessment for a possible **pneumothorax** should be performed.

▶ When possible, place the patient on a cardiac monitor to assist in identification of vagal stimulation. Some systems administer atropine, especially with younger patients, to prevent excessive vagal tone which causes bradycardia.

▶ The EDD is a quick and easy indicator of proper tube placement. Recent evidence suggests that the EDD is most accurate when used soon after intubation, before significant air is introduced. Excessive ventilation through a misplaced tube can result in a false-positive reading, making you believe you are in the trachea, when in fact, your tube is improperly placed in the esophagus.

▶ CASE STUDY

You and your partner are dispatched to a private residence for someone in cardiac arrest. When you approach the scene, you notice that there are several people standing in a huddle on the lawn. Assessing that the scene is safe, you approach and ask everyone to step back. In the middle of the huddle there is a 35-year-old female who is not moving or making any noise. She has circumoral cyanosis, and looks very pale. You assess for the ABCs and realize that she is not breathing, but she does have a slow pulse.

Your sympathetic nervous system kicks into overdrive as you instruct your partner to insert an appropriately sized OPA and begin BVM ventilations with 100 percent oxygen at a rate of 8-10 times per minute. The patient accepts the OPA, so you prepare your intubation equipment. You choose a 7.5 ETT, and check the cuff by attaching a 10-cc syringe and inflating it with air, leaving it in the packaging to prevent contamination. You deflate the cuff and insert a stylette to a level just above the Murphy's eye and form the tube into a "hockey stick" shape. You set the prepared ETT aside and make sure that the light on your laryngoscope is white, tight, and bright.

Knowing that you are about 30 seconds from your intubation attempt, you ask your partner to preoxygenate the patient, and ask her to take out and hold on to the OPA when you are ready to intubate. You make sure that the suction unit works and has a rigid-tip catheter attached to the suction tubing, then place it by the patient's right side, where you always look for it when needed. You give your partner the go-ahead nod, and she moves off to the patient's left while you move in from the right.

You open the patient's mouth with a scissor technique, and proceed to insert the Miller blade into the patient's mouth. You visualize that the blade is covering the epiglottis, so you lift up on the handle and lift the mandible out of the way until the whites of the vocal cords are visualized. You ask your partner for the ETT and place the tube so that the black indicator on the tube is right at the level of the vocal cords. An esophageal detector device placed on the end of the tube reinflates without difficulty. You inflate the ETT cuff, pull out the stylette, attach the BVM and colormetric $ETCO_2$ device, and begin to ventilate the patient. You visualize adequate chest rise and fall, and condensation begins to form in the tube. You grab for the stethoscope and auscultate for equal lung sounds and negative sounds over the epigastric. You confirm color change on the $ETCO_2$ detector, secure the tube using an aftermarket device, reassess lung sounds, and continue your exam. ■

CHAPTER 2

Endotracheal Tube Extubation

KEY TERMS

Aspiration

Aspiration pneumonia

Hypoxic

Left lateral position

OBJECTIVES

The student will be able to do the following:

▶ List the indications for performing endotracheal tube extubation in a patient (pp. 15–16).

▶ Describe the importance of properly performing endotracheal tube extubation (pp. 15–16).

▶ Describe the proper technique used when performing endotracheal extubation in a patient (pp. 16–18).

▶ Demonstrate the ability to properly perform endotracheal tube extubation (pp. 16–18).

INTRODUCTION

What happens if your patient begins to gag with an endotracheal tube (ETT) in place, or if the patient begins to have spontaneous respirations? These are two indications for immediate extubation. Extubation is the reverse of intubation, or the rapid removal of an ETT.

Two situations in which you may consider extubation include (1) the suspicion that an ETT has dislodged from the trachea and (2) significant patient improvement after successful treatment. Examples of patients who may require extubation after successful treatment include those who are unconscious or seizing from hypoglycemia but who become alert after administration of dextrose, those who overdose on narcotics and require early airway control but then respond favorably to treatment with naloxone, and post-cardiac arrest patients who respond to defibrillation.

In an unconscious patient suspected of having a misplaced or dislodged ETT, extubation is a fairly straightforward procedure. The oropharynx is suctioned, the cuff deflated, and the ETT removed from the patient. In a conscious and alert patient who has responded to treatment, the procedure is a bit more involved but still relatively easy and straightforward. This procedure will be detailed later in the chapter.

There are a couple of things that you need to do prior to extubating your patient. It is very important to lay the patient in a **left lateral position,** or sit them upright, and a suction unit with a rigid catheter should be turned on and ready for use, assuring that you can clear the pharynx of any secretions or emesis prior to deflating the ETT cuff, eliminating the possibility of aspiration.

When you are ready, suction the oropharynx, lay the patient in the left lateral position, deflate the cuff, and instruct the patient to take a deep breath. At the deepest part of the patient's inspiration, rapidly withdraw the ETT from the trachea while continuing to suction. As soon as the ETT is removed, place the patient on 100 percent oxygen via a nonrebreather mask, or at least administer blow-by oxygen for the patient if he is actively coughing or vomiting.

After the airway has been cleared and the patient is able to protect his own airway, you can sit the patient up and reassess him, and complete an initial and focused physical history and exam.

▶ EQUIPMENT

You will need the following equipment (Figure 2.1):

▶ Gloves
▶ Goggles
▶ Suction equipment
▶ Stethoscope
▶ 10-cc syringe
▶ High-flow, high-concentration oxygen source
▶ Nonrebreather mask

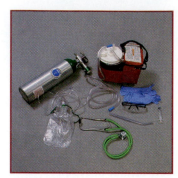

Figure 2.1

ASSESSMENT

Prior to removing an endotracheal tube, you should make sure that one of two situations exists, as evidenced by the clinical exam. One, that an intubated patient's ETT is not in the trachea, or two, that an intubated patient no longer requires the airway protection afforded by an ETT. Indications of displacement or esophageal intubation requiring immediate extubation include the absence of chest rise with ventilation, absence of breath sounds bilaterally, auscultation of air entering the epigastric region with ventilations, purple color indicator on the $ETCO_2$ detector in a patient with adequate perfusion, or a capnometry reading near zero. Indications for extubation after successful treatment (and all must be present) include the regaining of consciousness, unaltered mental status, spontaneous respirations with adequate rate and tidal volume, adequate SaO_2, and the patient gagging on or coughing around the ETT.

 ## PROCEDURE: Endotracheal Tube Extubation

1. Take infection control precautions.

Rationale: Gloves and goggles are used when working around the airway to ensure that infectious respiratory contents are not splashed into the rescuer's face.

 GERIATRIC NOTE:

Many geriatric patients have weakened immune systems and are more susceptible to respiratory infections. To prevent acquiring a respiratory illness from the patient, a mask may be indicated in addition to gloves and goggles.

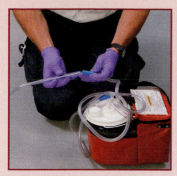
Figure 2.2

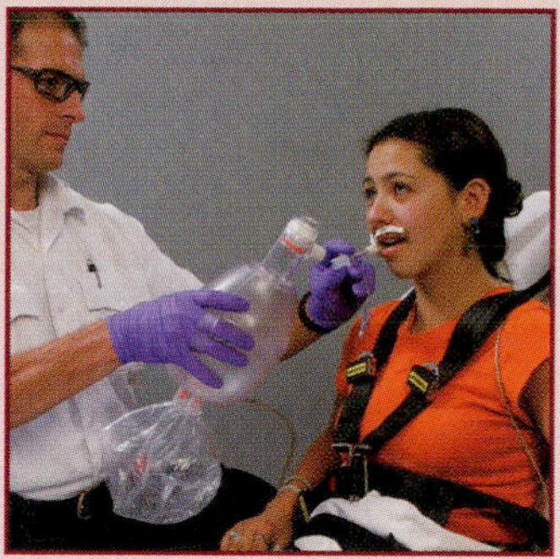

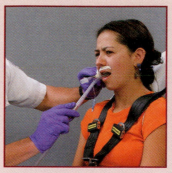
Figure 2.3

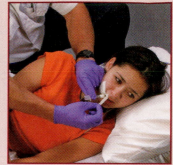
Figure 2.4

Figure 2.5

2. Assemble suction equipment and ensure suction is in working order (Figure 2.2).

   Rationale: Suction equipment must be charged or attached to a power source in order to suction strongly enough to remove airway contaminates such as sputum, blood, or vomit.

3. Explain the procedure to the patient (Figure 2.3).

   Rationale: Extubation nearly always causes the patient to cough, and sometimes to vomit. Prepare the patient for this temporary discomfort. In addition, you will need the patient to take a deep breath to assist in the procedure.

4. Suction the oropharynx (Figure 2.4).

   Rationale: Removing matter from the oropharynx will prevent the patient from aspirating should he or she inhale immediately upon removal of the endotracheal tube.

> **PEDIATRIC NOTE:**
>
> Remember that the oropharynx of a child or infant is much shorter than that of an adult. Be sure to measure the suction catheter from the corner of the mouth to the angle of the jaw and do not insert the catheter further than this distance into the mouth of the pediatric patient.

5. Place patient in the left lateral position.

   Rationale: Should the patient vomit upon removal of the tube, left lateral positioning will help prevent **aspiration**.

6. Remove any device that is securing the ETT (Figure 2.5).

   Rationale: Tape, or any other securing device, will need to be removed prior to extubation.

7. Completely deflate the distal cuff of the endotracheal tube using a 10-cc syringe (Figure 2.6).

   Rationale: If the cuff is not deflated, damage will occur to the trachea during removal of the tube.

> **PEDIATRIC NOTE:**
>
> If an uncuffed tube was used on the pediatric patient, then there will be no cuff to deflate. Typically, endotracheal tubes under size 5.5 will be uncuffed. Cuffed tracheal tubes are as safe as uncuffed tubes for infants (except newborns) and children if rescuers use the correct tube size and cuff inflation pressure and verify tube position. Under certain circumstances (eg., poor lung compliance, high airway resistance, and large glottic airleak), cuffed tracheal tubes may be preferable.

8. At the end of a deep inspiration, quickly remove the ETT while suctioning the oropharynx (Figure 2.7).

   Rationale: The sensation of extubation is uncomfortable, so it should be done carefully but quickly.

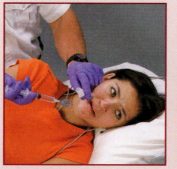
Figure 2.6

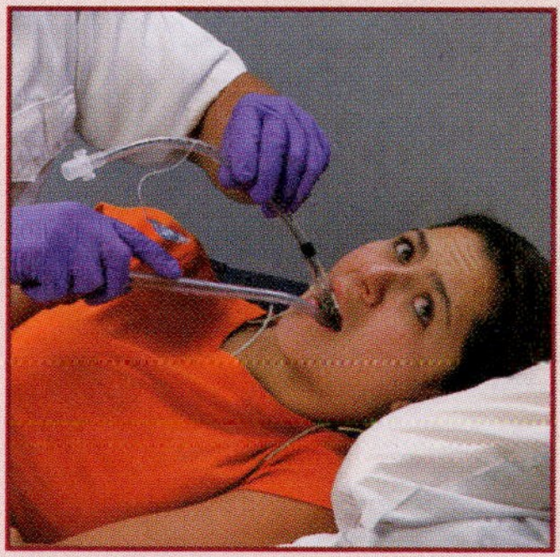

Figure 2.7

continued...

9. Sit the patient up, and ensure airway patency and adequate ventilatory status (Figure 2.8).

   Rationale: Even after a thorough assessment and determination to extubate, the patient may not begin breathing on his or her own. If adequate ventilatory status is not achieved immediately after extubation, consider assisting ventilations or re-intubating.

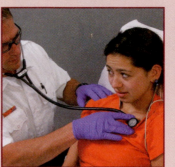 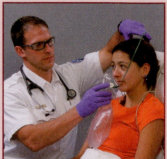

Figure 2.8   **Figure 2.9**

GERIATRIC NOTE:

Due to underlying disease processes, it is common for geriatric patients to have some difficulty regaining adequate respirations following extubation. If adequate rate and tidal volume are not achieved after several minutes following extubation, consider re-intubation.

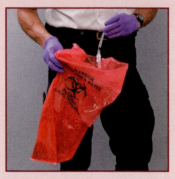

Figure 2.10

10. Place the patient on high-flow, high-concentration oxygen via nonrebreather face mask (Figure 2.9).

    Rationale: The suctioning and extubation may have made the patient **hypoxic.** Supplemental oxygen will help the patient regain adequate oxygenation levels.

11. Dispose of all equipment in a biohazard bag (Figure 2.10).

Rationale: Equipment that was used in or around the airway will be contaminated with potentially infectious material and must be disposed of in a biohazard container.

ONGOING ASSESSMENT

If the decision to extubate has been made, then by nature, it has been determined that the patient is improving and now able to manage his or her own airway. However, following the extubation procedure, it is possible that patients will not begin spontaneously breathing, or will not be able to maintain, over a period of time, adequate ventilation and oxygenation themselves. Therefore, constant monitoring of the airway and respiratory status is required. In fact, some systems prefer sedation to prehospital extubation.

In addition to all other elements of the ongoing assessment, such as heart rate, blood pressure, skin condition, and mental status, reassessment of airway patency, respiratory rate, tidal volume, and lung sounds are required. Should the patient begin to hypoventilate, consider assisting ventilations with a bag-valve mask or re-intubate as indicated.

It is not uncommon for the patient to experience throat pain, hoarseness, or difficulty swallowing post extubation. Difficulty swallowing carries with it an increased risk of aspiration, especially in the elderly patient. In addition, severe glottic edema may lead to post extubation stridor and obstruction. Developing stridor may be treated with nebulized racemic epinephrine, and the patient should be promptly re-intubated if you feel that a total airway obstruction is developing.

▶PROBLEM SOLVING

▶ The mortality rate with an **aspiration pneumonia** is extremely high. Be sure to suction adequately and avoid allowing the patient to inhale blood or vomit.

▶ Extubation will almost certainly stimulate the patient's gag reflex. Be sure to suction during extubation, not just before and after extubation.

▶ Suctioning during extubation can be difficult because one hand is on the tube to remove it and the other is holding the suction catheter. It may be necessary to employ the help of an assistant to suction for you while you concentrate on deflating the cuff and removing the tube.

▶ Instruct patients to take a deep breath during the procedure. This opens the vocal cords and often prevents gagging and subsequent vomiting during extubation.

▶CASE STUDY

You and your partner are transporting a patient after successfully reviving him from a witnessed cardiac arrest. As you are assessing for respirations and a pulse, you hear the faint sounds of the patient beginning to cough and gag. A few moments later, you note that the patient is tracking you and your partner with his eyes. You sit down next to him and begin to ask closed-ended questions that he can answer by nodding his head, and you are able to determine that he is alert and oriented. Your partner confirms that the patient's SaO_2 is 100 percent, $ETCO_2$ is 40 mmHg, and the patient's lungs are clear and his skin warm and dry. You note a normal sinus rhythm on the monitor, a pulse of 82 and regular, and a BP of 126/70.

After determining that his respiratory status will support extubation, you explain the procedure to the patient, and he nods that he understands. You suction his oropharynx, turn him on his left side, remove the tape securing the tube, and deflate the cuff. You instruct the patient to take a deep breath and pull the ETT out while continuing to suction. The patient coughs violently and regurgitates a bit of vomit into his mouth, which you promptly suction away. Once the vomit is clear from his airway, you roll the patient onto his back, then sit him up. The patient picks his head up as you place a nonrebreather oxygen mask on him and says "Thank you" in a hoarse voice. "You're welcome," you reply as you begin your reassessment. ■

CHAPTER 3

Pediatric ET Intubation

KEY TERMS

Bag-valve mask (BVM)

Cricoid pressure

Cuffed ETT

Hypercapnia

Hypoxemia

Macintosh blade

Miller blade

Nasopharyngeal airway

Oropharyngeal airway

Patent

Preoxygenation

Sellick's maneuver

Stylette

Uncuffed ETT

Vallecula

OBJECTIVES

The student will be able to do the following:

▶ List the indications for performing endotracheal intubation in the pediatric patient (pp. 20–25).

▶ Discuss the importance of properly performing endotracheal intubation in the pediatric patient (pp. 20–25).

▶ Describe the proper technique for performing endotracheal intubation in the pediatric patient (pp. 25–28).

▶ Demonstrate the ability to perform endotracheal intubation in the pediatric patient (pp. 25–28).

INTRODUCTION

As in the adult, endotracheal intubation (ETI) is the "gold standard" for obtaining a **patent** airway in the pediatric patient. Unlike adults, pediatric patients do not commonly go into cardiac arrest secondary to cardiac problems. Rather, cardiac arrest in the pediatric patient is most often a result of a precedent respiratory arrest. This places even more importance on control of the airway in the pediatric patient, as it will very often truly be a life-saving measure. Failure to adequately control the airway in the pediatric patient is very likely to result in death.

 PEDIATRIC NOTE:

Bag-valve mask ventilation can be as effective as ventilation through an endotracheal tube for short periods of time. In the prehospital setting ventilate and oxygenate infants and children with a bag-valve mask device, especially if transport time is short (class IIa recommendation).

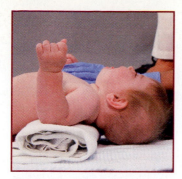

Figure 3.1

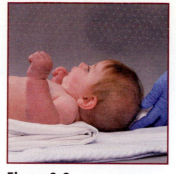

Figure 3.2

The advantages and indications for pediatric intubation mirror those of the adult (see Chapter 1) and also include the need for tracheal suctioning in the neonate during instances of meconium aspiration. There are no direct contraindications for intubation of the pediatric patient. While endotracheal intubation of both the pediatric and adult patient follow the same basic procedures, the pediatric airway differs from the adult's in several significant anatomic and physiologic ways, resulting in specific clinical consequences that should be of concern to you.

The airway of the pediatric patient is much smaller in length and diameter than an adult's, and can be easily kinked and occluded if the patient's neck becomes hyperextended (Figure 3.1) in an attempt to open the airway, or hyperflexed (Figure 3.2) if the airway is neglected. In addition, a relatively small amount of edema, caused by disease or injury from repeated intubation attempts, can result in a significant reduction in airflow and a decrease in airway compliance and increased work of breathing.

The tongue of the pediatric patient is larger relative to the oropharynx, and pediatric patients produce more oral secretions compared to an adult. Both of these situations can make airway control more difficult for you. Anterior displacement of the large tongue and copious secretions can interfere with BLS ventilation as well as make intubation difficult. These difficulties can be easily overcome by using an appropriately sized **oro-** or **nasopharyngeal airway** and aggressively suctioning the pediatric patient as needed.

The more anterior and superior position of the pediatric larynx, along with a larger tongue, can make visualization of the glottic opening difficult. Utilizing a **Miller blade** for your ETI attempt can compensate for this situation, as it affords slightly more epiglottic displacement than the **Macintosh blade**.

The epiglottis in infants and toddlers tends to be more narrow, floppy, and longer than in adults. The vocal cords have a different appearance (they tend to be less white) and attach more anteriorly than an adult's. Again, a Miller blade may be of more benefit than a Macintosh, as it is designed to lift the epiglottis and will remove it from your line of sight to the glottis. You must be familiar with the differences in anatomy appearance in the pediatric patient so you can identify specific airway landmarks such as the epiglottis, arytenoid cartilage, and glottic opening.

In younger pediatric patients, the narrowest part of the airway is not the vocal cords, as in an adult, but at the level of the cricoid ring, which will "grip" the

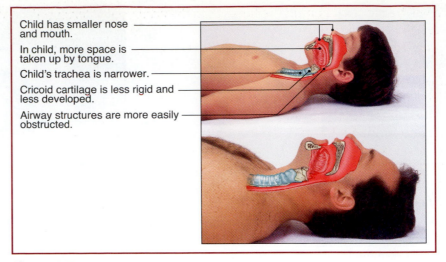

Child has smaller nose and mouth.
In child, more space is taken up by tongue.
Child's trachea is narrower.
Cricoid cartilage is less rigid and less developed.
Airway structures are more easily obstructed.

Figure 3.3

endotracheal tube and act as a "physiological cuff" (Figure 3.3). As a result, the ETT is sized for the cricoid ring, not the glottis, and an **uncuffed ETT** is used. To aid in proper depth insertion, most pediatric ETTs have a vocal cord marker at the distal one third of the tube (Figure 3.4). The ETT should be inserted to a depth that places this marker between the vocal cords. In addition, some use the formula: depth of insertion (cm) = (age in years ÷ 2) + 12.

The use of a length-based resuscitation tape (see Chapter 25), such as the Broselow® tape (Figure 3.5), is recommended for determining ETT size in the pediatric patient. In addition, the formula: uncuffed tube size = (age in years ÷ 4) + 4 may be used to determine the appropriately sized uncuffed ETT. If a **cuffed ETT** will be used, the formula: cuffed tube size = (age in years ÷ 4) + 3 may be used to determine the appropriately sized ETT.

As in the adult, one of our goals is to open the pediatric patient's airway and place him in the "sniffing" position, with the ear canal at the same level as the sternal notch. This position aligns the oral, pharyngeal, and tracheal axis, allowing for better visualization of the glottis. How this is achieved, however, differs according to the physical development and anatomical characteristics of each pediatric patient. Newborns and infants, because of their large heads in relation to their bodies, require padding under their shoulders to prevent hyperflexion of their necks and resultant airway occlusion (Figure 3.6). As it happens, the combination of large occiput and padding below the shoulders sometimes creates the exact head elevation desired for optimal airway control and laryngeal visualization during ETI, making padding beneath the head unnecessary. For children older than 2 years old,

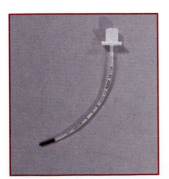

Figure 3.4

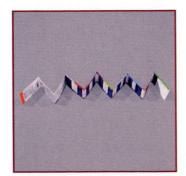

Figure 3.5

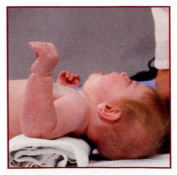

Figure 3.6

padding will be required behind the head, as in the adult, but often significantly less than is required for the adult.

After placing the patient in the proper position, preoxygenation by BLS ventilation utilizing an oro- or nasopharyngeal airway, **bag-valve mask (BVM)**, and 100 percent oxygen should precede ETI. Tidal volume delivered with each ventilation should be sufficient to result in normal rise and fall of the chest. As it is admittedly difficult to memorize all of the particulars for all age groups and expect to have perfect recall during an understandably stressful time, it is strongly recommended that you carry some sort of reference chart on your person to provide you with these parameters.

The use of a pulse oximeter can help with assessing **preoxygenation** in patients with a pulse. Individuals providing BLS airway control should attempt to achieve a SaO_2 as close to 100 percent as possible. In all patients, evaluation of chest rise and fall, mask seal, BVM compliance, and patient color will be a better indication of the effectiveness of ventilations. In **Sellick's maneuver**, pressure is placed on the cricoid cartilage during positive-pressure ventilation, compressing the esophagus. This reduces gastric distension and passive regurgitation and helps bring the vocal cords into view, which is useful if intubation is to be performed (Figure 3.7).

Care must be taken not to press with so much pressure that the fragile trachea is occluded. Ensure the patient is well oxygenated before attempting intubation.

Again, for all of the differences in the pediatric patient, ETI in the pediatric patient follows the same procedures as in the adult. The patient must be adequately preoxygenated prior to the intubation attempt, and the attempt should be stopped and BVM ventilations resumed when the SaO_2 drops to 90 percent in a perfusing patient, or after 30 seconds in a patient in cardiac arrest. It is important to remember that the pediatric patient will desaturate faster than an adult, requiring particular attention to SaO_2 in patients with a pulse.

Pediatric patients are at high risk for ET tube misplacement, displacement, or obstruction. Correct ETT placement should be confirmed immediately after intubation, after securing the ETT with tape or a secure device, during transport, and any time the patient is moved. Endotracheal placement of the tube should be confirmed by both primary as well as a secondary means. Primary means include assessing clinical signs such as chest rise and fall, bilateral lung sounds, and absence of epigastric sounds. Exhaled CO_2 sensors and the esophageal detector device (EDD) are secondary means used to verify proper ET tube placement.

Regardless of the treatment setting, (i.e. prehospital, emergency departments, or operating rooms), CO_2 colorimetric detectors or capnometry should be used to

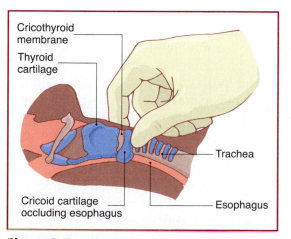

Cricothyroid membrane

Thyroid cartilage

Trachea

Cricoid cartilage occluding esophagus

Esophagus

Figure 3.7

confirm tracheal tube placement in all intubated infants and children with a perfusing cardiac rhythm. Exhaled CO_2 may be difficult to detect during a cardiac arrest, therefore ETT placement should be confirmed using direct laryngoscopy.

The esophageal detector device is a self-inflating bulb that fits on the end of the ETT following intubation. It may be used to confirm ET tube placement for children weighing greater > 20 kg. $ETCO_2$ detectors are not recommended in infants weighing less than 2 kg. Due to the lack of an inflatable cuff, extra care must be taken to secure the ETT with tape or a commercial device, especially if an $ETCO_2$ detector is used, as it adds weight to the proximal ETT and increases the risk of dislodgement.

► EQUIPMENT

You will need the following equipment (Figure 3.8):

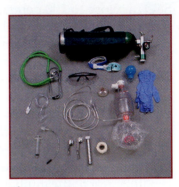

Figure 3.8

- ► Gloves
- ► Goggles
- ► Face mask
- ► Length-based resuscitation tape
- ► Suction equipment
- ► Endotracheal tubes (various sizes)
- ► Stylette
- ► Laryngoscope handle (with working batteries)
- ► Laryngoscope blades (various sizes and types)
- ► Stethoscope
- ► Bag-valve mask
- ► Tape or commercial tube securing device
- ► Esophageal detector device
- ► Colormetric $ETCO_2$ detector (or other $ETCO_2$ device)

► ASSESSMENT

While ETI is considered an ALS skill, the assessment of a patient requiring intubation focuses on the basics: airway, breathing, and circulation (ABCs). The most obvious assessment finding that should result in an immediate attempt to intubate is apnea secondary to respiratory or cardiac arrest. In addition, severe respiratory distress, as evidenced by tachypnea, tachycardia, nasal flaring, grunting, retractions, peripheral cyanosis, and anxiety, can quickly lead to respiratory failure and arrest.

Respiratory distress will commonly respond to supplemental oxygen administration and not require intubation, but signs and symptoms of respiratory failure strongly suggests the need for ETI. These signs and symptoms include poor muscle tone, tachycardia deteriorating to bradycardia, tachypnea deteriorating to bradypnea, central cyanosis, and lethargy. It is important to remember that the progression from respiratory distress to respiratory failure to respiratory and then cardiac arrest can occur quickly, requiring that you assess the patient frequently and secure the airway, oxygenate, and ventilate early.

Impending airway obstruction requiring ETI can be anticipated by recognizing the potential for the development of obstruction exists. Patients with airway burns, anaphylaxis, or epiglottitis should be considered at high risk for the development of airway obstruction and monitored closely for the development or worsening of dysphagia, drooling, a hoarse voice, stridor, and respiratory distress. Remember that a small amount of edema or swelling can significantly reduce the diameter of the narrow pediatric airway. Therefore, it is especially important to recognize the signs and symptoms early, have your ETI equipment prepared, and make the decision to intubate prior to total occlusion. Foreign body airway obstruction (FBAO), as evidenced by apnea, cyanosis, loss of consciousness, and inability to ventilate, requires immediate foreign body removal under direct laryngoscopy. Toddlers are at high risk for FBAO because they tend to place things in their mouths.

Unconsciousness, in and of itself, is not an absolute indication for ETI, but is when combined with a lack of a gag reflex and a risk of aspiration. As most patients in the prehospital environment can be assumed to have some gastric content, any patient you encounter without a gag reflex is a strong candidate for ETI. Certainly, if your patient accepts an OPA and is receiving positive-pressure ventilations, ETI is indicated unless you expect rapid improvement in the patient's condition, such as a hypoglycemic patient who is about to receive dextrose or a toddler who has just had a FBAO removed and can be expected to respond to ventilation and oxygenation. If these patients are vomiting and the airway is uncontrollable, however, immediate intubation may be required.

Deep tracheal suctioning to treat meconium aspiration is also an indication for ETI in the newborn. Meconium-stained, depressed infants should receive tracheal suctioning immediately after birth and before stimulation, presuming the equipment and expertise is available. Tracheal suctioning is not necessary for babies with meconium-stained fluid who are vigorous. The presence of thick versus thin meconium should not determine whether you perform these skills; the clinical condition of your patient should. Signs and symptoms of newborn depression include bradypnea, weak respiratory effort, grunting, lack of a strong cry, poor muscle tone, bradycardia, and cyanosis unresponsive to oxygenation.

PROCEDURE: Pediatric ET Intubation

1. Prepare the pediatric patient for intubation. If the child has a perfusing rhythm, place the child on an O_2 saturation, cardiorespiratory, and blood pressure monitor prior to intubation and monitor continuously during the intubation attempt.

   Rationale: Monitoring the patient's O_2 saturation and heart rate will alert you early if the patient's condition begins to deteriorate secondary to hypoxemia. Bradycardia, cyanosis, and pallor are clinical signs of hypoxemia.

2. Prepare equipment, medications, and personnel prior to the intubation attempt. Prepare and confirm working condition of all intubation equipment and have it readily accessible for the procedure. Prepare all pre-procedure medications based on the child's weight and height and have them ready for administration. This would include all medications for rapid sequence intubation (RSI) if indicated, including cardiovascular adjuncts such as atropine,

   sedative-hypnotic agents such as etomidate or Versed, anesthetic agents such as lidocaine, and neuromuscular blocking agents such as succinylcholine or vecuonium. You will need to refer to your local protocols for the approved medications for this procedure.

   Rationale: Medications for RSI are administered to minimize the potentially dangerous physiologic responses that can occur with intubation including profound vagal stimulation resulting in bradycardia, tachycardia, hypertension, increased intracranial pressure, and laryngospasm.

3. Take infection control precautions.

   Rationale: Gloves, goggles, and a face mask are essential equipment when working around the airway since infectious diseases are transmitted through airway secretions.

continued...

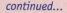

4. Open the airway manually with either the head tilt-chin lift with head elevation technique (Figure 3.9) or jaw thrust (Figure 3.10) for trauma victims. Depending on the age of the patient, padding may need to be placed under the shoulders or head to achieve this position.

   Rationale: Proper positioning of the airway will assist the rescuer in removing the tongue as an airway obstruction, providing more adequate BVM ventilations, and visualizing the cords during endotracheal intubation. The large head of infants and toddlers may require padding under the shoulders, while a child may require padding under the head.

5. Ensure the gag reflex is absent, and elevate the tongue with a simple airway adjunct such as an oropharyngeal airway (Figure 3.11).

   Rationale: When ventilating the non-intubated patient, an airway adjunct helps to remove the tongue as an airway obstruction. In addition, it helps assess for the presence of a gag reflex.

6. Begin ventilating the patient with an appropriately sized BVM attached to 100 percent oxygen at a rate appropriate for the patient's age (Figure 3.12).

   Rationale: The patient is presumably hypoxemic and/or hypercapnic, and ventilation will help to correct these conditions. While room air delivers an oxygen concentration of 21 percent, high-flow high-concentration oxygen via BVM will deliver at least 85 percent oxygen concentration, which can correct **hypoxemia** and **hypercapnia** quicker. Use of an appropriately sized BVM helps reduce the risk of providing too much tidal volume and causing barotrauma.

7. Apply **cricoid pressure** (patients older than 1 year), and continue ventilating at a rate appropriate for the patient's age with enough tidal volume to achieve normal chest rise.

   Rationale: Ventilation at a rate appropriate for the patient's age prevents blowing off too much carbon dioxide, which is dangerous because it causes vasoconstriction. Generally speaking, provide 12-20 ventilations per minute to an apneic child with a perfusing rhythm and 8-10 breaths per minute for a child receiving CPR. Ventilation volumes adequate to produce normal chest rise and fall are desirable to prevent

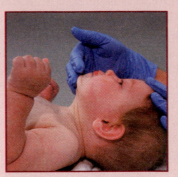
Figure 3.9

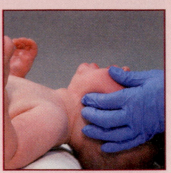
Figure 3.10

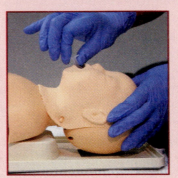
Figure 3.11

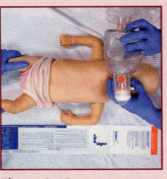
Figure 3.12

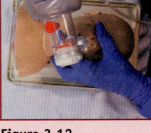
Figure 3.13

complications such as gastric insufflation, barotrauma, and decreased venous return to the heart. Cricoid pressure helps to reduce gastric insufflation and passive regurgitation.

8. Select the proper equipment for intubation, including a properly sized laryngoscope blade, endotracheal tube and stylette, and tape or tube securing device. A length-based resuscitation tape can be used to determine proper equipment size (see Chapter 25) (Figure 3.13).

   Rationale: Many types and sizes of equipment exist. Selecting properly sized equipment will help ensure successful tube placement.

9. Insert a **stylette** into the ETT to a depth about 2 cm below the distal end, just below the Murphy's eye (Figure 3.14).

   Rationale: The stylette will provide rigidity to the ETT, and proper insertion depth is necessary to prevent injury to the airway.

10. Check the laryngoscope and light bulb by assembling the handle and blade combination to ensure the light comes on, is white and bright, and cannot be easily unscrewed from its position (Figure 3.15).

    Rationale: An improperly functioning laryngoscope will make it difficult to visualize the cords and pass the ETT.

11. Ventilate the patient with 100 percent O_2 via a bag-valve mask device to achieve an O_2 saturation near or at 100 percent. The exact rate will depend on the patient's age. Avoid aggressive positive-pressure ventilation.

    Rationale: Ventilation will not take place during the intubation attempt. Aggressive positive-pressure ventilation may cause gastric inflation, increasing the risk of aspiration.

12. Remove the previously inserted airway adjunct (Figure 3.16).

    Rationale: Since the tongue of a child is so large, it will be easier to visualize the cords with no obstacles in the mouth.

13. Open the patient's mouth using the "scissor" technique.

    Rationale: The scissor technique allows you to open the patient's mouth without inserting your fingers and risking a bite injury.

14. Hold the laryngoscope in your left hand, insert the laryngoscope blade on the right side of the mouth, and move it toward the left to displace the tongue (Figure 3.17).

    Rationale: Displacing the tongue to the left prevents it from obstructing your view of the vocal cords.

15. With the tip of the laryngoscope, follow the tongue into the hypopharynx, identify the epiglottis, and, if using a Miller blade, lift the epiglottis. If using a Macintosh blade, insert the tip into the **vallecula**.

    Rationale: Each blade is designed to be used in a specific fashion. Use of the Miller blade is recommended in pediatric patients as it allows better lift of the epiglottis and visualization of the glottis.

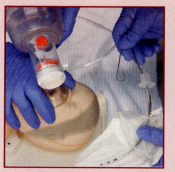

Figure 3.14

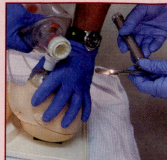

Figure 3.15

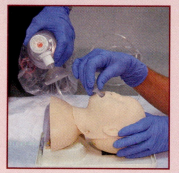

Figure 3.16

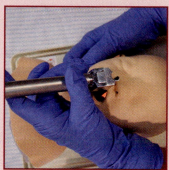

Figure 3.17

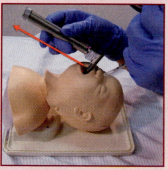

Figure 3.18

16. Lifting upward along the axis of the laryngoscope handle and without flexing your wrist, elevate the mandible with the laryngoscope blade and visualize the vocal cords (Figure 3.18).

    Rationale: Elevating the mandible by lifting the laryngoscope allows visual access of the cords. Flexing your wrist will not elevate the mandible, but will put pressure on the teeth, potentially breaking them. If the mandible is not displaced well enough or far enough, the cords will remain obscured and no tube can be placed.

17. Introduce the ET tube while maintaining direct visualization of the vocal cords. Advance to the

continued...

proper depth as indicated by markings on the pediatric ETT (Figure 3.19a, Figure 3.19b).

Rationale: A tube inserted too far will likely end up in the mainstem bronchus, allowing only one lung to be inflated.

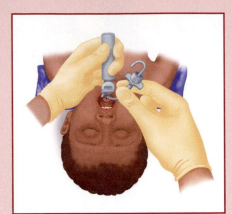

Figure 3.19a

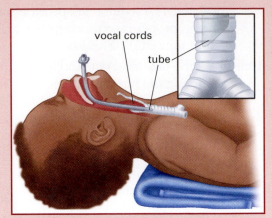

Figure 3.19b

18. Remove the stylette from the ETT (Figure 3.20), and use an esophageal detector device to confirm tracheal placement of the tube in children weighing 20 kg with a perfusing cardiac rhythm (Figure 3.21).

Rationale: Utilization of an esophageal detector device aids in identifying esophageal intubations. In infants and children with a perfusing rhythm, use a colorimetric detector or capnography to detect exhaled CO_2 to confirm endotracheal tube position in the prehospital and inhospital settings.

19. Confirm proper tube placement by auscultating for lung sounds bilaterally over each lung (Figure 3.22) and for the absence of sounds over the epigastrium (Figure 3.23). If no lung sounds are heard, extubation should be considered (see Chapter 2).

Rationale: Bilateral lung sounds are a primary indicator of proper tube placement.

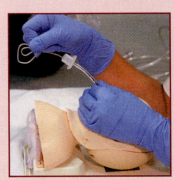

Figure 3.20

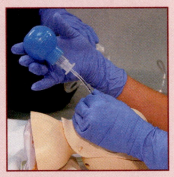

Figure 3.21

20. Direct ventilation of the patient while still manually securing the tube in place. Utilize an end-tidal carbon dioxide ($ETCO_2$) detector between the BVM and ETT to aid in confirmation of tracheal placement of the ETT.

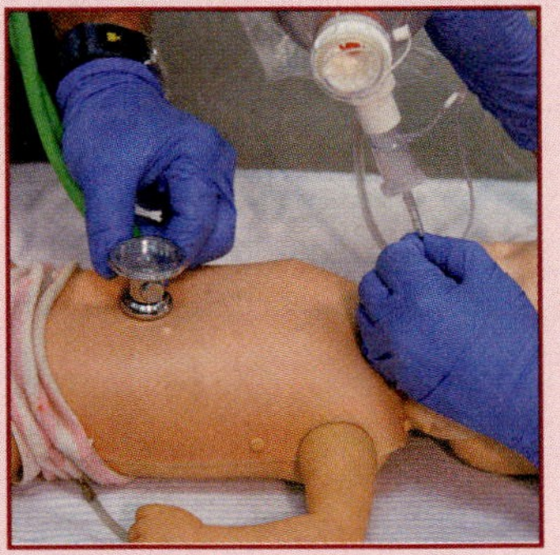

Rationale: Confirmation of tracheal placement of the ETT and ventilation should be initiated as quickly as possible.

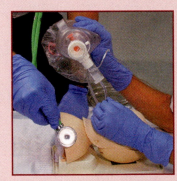

Figure 3.22

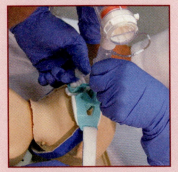

Figure 3.23

21. Secure the ETT with tape or a commercial securing device (Figure 3.24) and maintain the child's head in a neutral position following tube placement.

Rationale: A tube that is not properly secured may be dislodged. Head extension can displace the tube and pull it out of the airway or into the espohagus. Neck flexion may push the tube into a mainstem bronchus. All of which are life-threatening complications.

Figure 3.24

Many pediatric respiratory and cardiac arrests are related to underlying respiratory illnesses or diseases. Frequent reassessment of the respiratory status, including rate, effort, and lung sounds, is indicated for the intubated child. However, reassessment of vital signs and mental status is equally important.

Reassessment of tube placement is a key to prevent accidental dislodgement of the tube into the esophagus, which is life-threatening. Because pediatric ET tubes maybe uncuffed and very pliable, they are easily dislodged during ventilation and transport. Frequent reassessment of lung sounds, absence of epigastric sounds, condensation in the tube, chest rise, skin color, capnometry, and even pulse oximetry can help confirm that the tube remains in the trachea.

▶ PROBLEM SOLVING

▶ If secretions, fluid, or food exist in the airway and prevent visualization of the cords, suction prior to making any intubation attempts.

▶ Be sure not to use the teeth as a fulcrum, even in children who do not yet have their permanent teeth. Using the laryngoscope in a manner against its intended design will not result in better visualization, and can be harmful to the patient.

▶ A properly sized pediatric ventilation bag is essential to ensure that excessive volumes of air are not introduced into the lungs, causing barotrauma. Ventilation bags and bag-mask devices come in many sizes, from neonate to toddler. If forced to use a ventilation bag that is too large, use only one hand to squeeze the bag, and do not squeeze the bag fully.

▶ CASE STUDY

You and your partner are dispatched to a local swimming pool where you find a 5-year-old male lying next to the pool face down, surrounded by a concerned crowd of people. A firefighter from the responding engine company provides c-spine stabilization as the other firefighters secure the scene by moving the crowd back. On the firefighter's command, you and your partner assist in rolling the patient into a supine position. You assess for respirations, and determine that the child is not breathing. You feel for and detect a fast, regular brachial pulse. The child has circumoral cyanosis and is cold to the touch.

Your partner inserts an OPA and begins BVM ventilations with 100 percent oxygen while you prepare for ET intubation. Your partner directs one of the other firefighters to apply the pulse oximeter and then provide cricoid pressure while he continues to ventilate. You prepare your equipment, place the suction unit by the patient's head as you move over to the patient. As he removes the BVM and takes the OPA out of the patient's mouth, you note a SaO_2 of 100 percent. You open the patient's mouth with a scissor technique, insert the laryngoscope, and lift the mandible. You immediately note and suction the secretions that have collected in the patient's hypopharynx, then lift the epiglottis with the Miller blade. The glottic opening immediately comes into view and you pass the ETT through the vocal cords.

You pull the laryngoscope out of the patient's mouth while holding the ETT at the patient's lip, then rule out esophageal intubation with a bulb-type esophageal detector device and apply the colormetric $ETCO_2$ detector. You direct your partner to resume ventilations as you see equal chest rise and fall, note condensation in the ETT, hear bilateral lung sounds, and hear nothing over the epigastric region. You look up and see color change from purple to yellow on the $ETCO_2$ detector and give your partner the thumbs up. Your capnometry reading is initially 55 mmHg, but quickly comes down to 40 mmHg. "We're in," you say, and begin to complete your assessment as a firefighter arrives with the immobilization gear. ■

CHAPTER 4

Suctioning through an Endotracheal Tube

KEY TERMS

Carina

Endotracheal (ET) tube

Hypoxia

Soft-tip suction catheter

OBJECTIVES

The student will be able to do the following:

▶ List the indications for performing suctioning through an endotracheal tube (pp. 30–31).

▶ Describe the importance of properly performing suctioning through an endotracheal tube (pp. 30–31).

▶ Describe the proper technique for performing suctioning through an endotracheal tube (pp. 31–33).

▶ Demonstrate the ability to perform suctioning through an endotracheal tube (pp. 31–35).

INTRODUCTION

Suctioning through an **endotracheal (ET) tube** is necessary in both medical and trauma patients. The goal is to clear the airway of unwanted material, vomit, blood, and other secretions. A **soft-tip suction catheter** is inserted down the ET tube to the level of the **carina**, the branching point of the trachea. A soft-tip suction catheter is a flexible, hollow plastic or rubber catheter that has a hard plastic adapter located on the proximal end. In addition to allowing connection to the suction tubing, a suction control hole in the adapter must be covered with the user's thumb to create suction at the distal tip of the catheter.

Suctioning is indicated when you identify fluids or other material in the endotracheal tube or airway. Potential complications of suctioning include tracheal trauma, increased ICP, hypoxial arrhythmias, and bradycardia. Patients frequently report that tracheal suctioning is extremely uncomfortable. Another potential complication of suctioning is the development of hypoxia during the procedure, the risk of which can be lessened by ventilating the patient, preceding and following suction attempts, with 100 percent oxygen. The suction attempt should not exceed 10-15 seconds. One to two mL of sterile saline may be instilled into the airway and dispersed with a few ventilations prior to suctioning. This will aid the suctioning removal of thick mucus, fluid, and other material in the airway. For diagnostic information on oxygenation status during suctioning, a pulse oximeter can be utilized, and the suction attempt stopped when the patient's SaO_2 falls to 90 percent.

Proper depth of insertion, to the level of the carina, needs to be assured to prevent too deep of an insertion and injury to the lung parenchyma. To determine the proper insertion depth, hold the distal tip of the catheter between your fingers at the nipple line and measure to the patient's ear, then from the ear to the tip of the endotracheal tube (ETT). Mark this point on the suction catheter with tape to easily identify it during the catheter insertion. As with the oropharynx, the suction catheter is inserted into the ETT to the predetermined level, then suction is applied while withdrawing the catheter. Suctioning efficacy can be improved by rolling the catheter between your fingers while withdrawing. To prevent extremely viscous mucus from obstructing the narrow lumen of the suction catheter, sterile water can be suctioned through the catheter between suctioning attempts to keep it clear of obstructions.

As endotracheal intubation bypasses the normal protective functions of the upper airway, aseptic technique should be utilized to ensure that you do not introduce bacteria into the lower airway during the suction attempt. The use of sterile gloves, not letting the suction catheter come into contact with nonsterile surfaces, and placing the catheter back in its sterile wrapper between suction attempts are all ways to help decrease the risk of infection.

▶EQUIPMENT

You will need the following equipment:

- ▶ Sterile gloves
- ▶ Goggles
- ▶ Suction unit
- ▶ Soft-tip suction catheter
- ▶ Sterile water

ASSESSMENT

You will know that the patient needs suctioning if you hear gurgling sounds coming from the ET tube, and you may visualize material, vomit, blood, or secretion accumulation in the ET tube as well. In addition, auscultation of the trachea and mainstem bronchi may reveal gurgling or rhonchi, indicating the presence of fluid or mucus in the airway.

PROCEDURE: Suctioning Through an Endotracheal Tube

1. Apply BSI precautions.

   Rationale: Gloves and eye protection are required at a minimum, and a gown may be needed if large amounts of blood or fluid are present to prevent exposure to infectious diseases.

2. Patient should be in a supine position.

   Rationale: Although the patient can be suctioned in other positions, supine is the recommended position.

3. Check and assemble equipment. Apply a new, sterile glove to the dominant hand.

   Rationale: You don't want to be in a position to suction and find the equipment does not work. Care should be taken during suctioning to ensure the newly gloved hand and suction catheter remain sterile to reduce the risk of contamination and introduction of infection to the airway.

continued...

4. Turn on the suction, being sure to keep the dominant hand sterile. If electric suction is being used, place the control on the lower suction pressure. If your suction unit has a gauge, set it between 80 and 120 mm.

   Rationale: Suction at higher pressures can cause damage to the airway if the suction tip goes beyond the ET tube.

5. Ventilate the patient prior to suctioning with 100 percent O_2. For thick secretions, blood or other material, consider instilling 1-2 mL of sterile saline and bag-mask ventilating the patient a few times before suctioning.

   Rationale: Patients can get hypoxic during the suctioning procedure. Sterile saline will thin secretions and facilitate successful suctioning. Disperse saline through the airways with positive pressure ventilation for maximal effect.

6. Measure the distance the catheter will be advanced. Measure the distance from the nipple line to the patient's ear (Figure 4.1), then from the ear to the top of the endotracheal tube (Figure 4.2). Place a piece of tape at that point. This should be just at or slightly beyond (1-2 cm) to the end of the ET tube.

   Rationale: Measuring the distance ensures that the suction tip will not go below the carina, causing airway damage and complications.

7. Using the sterile gloved hand, place the soft-tip suction catheter into the ET tube (Figure 4.3).

   Rationale: Care should be taken during suctioning that the gloved hand remains sterile. A sterile gloved hand reduces the risk of contamination of the suction catheter. Contamination of the suction catheter can cause introduction of infection into the airway.

8. Advance the catheter slowly down the ET tube (Figure 4.4) without applying the suction.

   Rationale: Fast insertion can increase the risk of gag and cough reflexes in the patient. As you suction you are removing oxygen from the respiratory system; therefore suction should only be applied while the catheter is on the way out of the ET tube.

9. When the catheter has been advanced to the proper distance, place your thumb over the

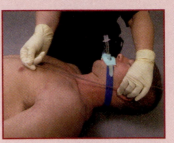

Figure 4.1

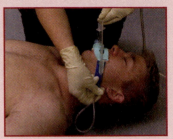

Figure 4.2

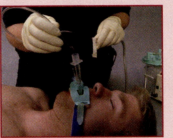

Figure 4.3

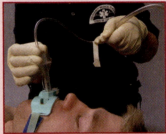

Figure 4.4

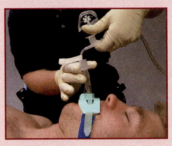

Figure 4.5

suction control hole and slowly withdraw the catheter while rotating or twisting the catheter between your fingers. Never suction for more than 10-15 seconds (Figure 4.5).

Rationale: Overinsertion of the catheter can cause injury to the airway. Placing your finger over the suction control hole allows suctioning to begin; rotating the catheter between your fingers increases the sweep of the catheter, allowing more material to be suctioned. Suctioning for more than 10 seconds can cause **hypoxia**.

10. Clean the catheter in sterile water to remove materials and/or fluids: Usually, a small amount of sterile saline is poured into the small box shaped dish that is included in the sterile suction

catheter kit. The catheter tip is then inserted into the dish to clear any debris. Sticking the catheter into the entire 500-1000 cc bottle of sterile saline/water will potentially introduce debris into the bottle making it unuseable for future suctioning attempts. (Figure 4.6).

Rationale: In most cases the suction catheter will become clogged with material. Cleaning the catheter keeps it clear.

11. When setting the catheter down, make sure it is placed in a sterile environment.

    Rationale: A sterile environment reduces the risk of contamination of the suction catheter. Contamination of the suction catheter can cause introduction of bacteria into the airway.

12. Ventilate the patient with 100 percent O$_2$ and repeat the procedure if necessary. Reglove if more suctioning is necessary.

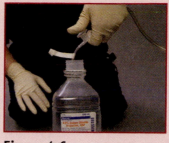

Figure 4.6

Rationale: Patients can become hypoxic during suctioning; ventilation reduces this risk. Regloving reduces the risk of introducing bacteria into the airway.

13. Document the procedure and outcome.

    Rationale: It is extremely important to document your findings in order to have a history of facts and events that occurred during patient care.

ONGOING ASSESSMENT

Assess the patient immediately after suctioning for signs of hypoxia. Constantly monitor the patient's need for repeat suctioning.

▶ PROBLEM SOLVING

▶ Hypoxia can result if the suctioning procedure takes too long. Good preoxygenation and monitoring of the time it takes to do the procedure can eliminate the onset of hypoxia.

▶ If you do not measure the suction catheter and advance it too far, you can cause the coughing reflex, bronchospasms, arrhythmias, and injury to the mucosa of the lower airways.

▶ Suction pressure that is too high can also cause the preceding complications. Monitor the pressure you are using.

▶ If the catheter becomes clogged with materials, place the tip of the soft-tip suction catheter into sterile water, put your thumb over the suction control hole, and draw water through the catheter. This will clear the catheter.

▶ If possible, place the patient on the cardiac monitor to assist in identification of excessive vagal stimulation and resultant bradycardia.

▶ Monitor the patient's oxygen saturation, heart rate, and general appearance throughout the suctioning procedure. If bradycardia develops or if the patient's oxygen saturation falls below 90 percent, suctioning should be immediately discontinued. Bradycardia and falling O$_2$ saturation are clinical signs of hypoxia, and a deteriorating patient condition. Terminating suctioning and ventilating the patient with 100 percent O$_2$ should improve the patient's condition.

▶ CASE STUDY

You are transporting a 43-year-old male who was involved in a single-car motor vehicle collision. The patient is unconscious and has massive facial trauma. While en route, your paramedic partner intubates the patient orally and advises you that the patient's airway was full of blood. She states that she is concerned that the patient still has blood in his airway.

As you begin to ventilate the patient, you note that ventilations are more difficult than usual. You report this difficulty to your partner. She auscultates for lung sounds and determines that the patient has equal sounds bilaterally. Your partner decides that since your transport time to the closest facility is still 15 minutes, she would like you to suction the patient's airway to help clear the ET tube to facilitate better ventilation of the patient. You prepare your equipment and don your eye shield and face mask.

You ask your partner to ventilate the patient and, after she has done so, the bag-valve device is removed from the end of the ET tube and you slowly insert the suction catheter through the end of the ET tube. Once you have reached your pre-measured depth, you cover the hole on the catheter with your thumb to apply suction. As you apply suction, you note that large amounts of bloody fluid are being removed from the patient's airway. After you complete suctioning of the patient, you ask your partner to hyperventilate the patient again. While she is ventilating the patient, she notes greater ease in bag compression. The patient is transported to the emergency department without further need for suctioning. ■

CHAPTER 5

Nasotracheal Intubation

OBJECTIVES

The student will be able to do the following:

▶ List the indications for performing nasotracheal intubation (pp. 35–38).

▶ Value the importance of properly performing nasotracheal intubation (pp. 35–38).

▶ Describe the proper technique for performing nasotracheal intubation (pp. 38–40).

▶ Demonstrate the ability in performing nasotracheal intubation (pp. 38–40).

INTRODUCTION

Nasotracheal intubation is an impressive airway intervention that can be used to obtain an adequate airway. Unlike all other methods of intubation, this skill requires that the patient be breathing spontaneously, and can be performed on either a conscious or unconscious patient. The primary indication for nasotracheal intubation is the need for advanced airway control when the inability to intubate orally exists. Oral intubation may be impossible due to oral trauma, significant **angioedema**, a conscious patient's intact gag reflex, or **trismus**. Possible spinal injury is another indication for the procedure, as it does not require manipulation of the cervical spine, like orotracheal intubation.

Contraindications for nasotracheal intubation include apnea, foreign body airway obstruction, severe facial injury, basilar skull fracture, the presence of a deviated septum or nasal obstruction, and a history of a bleeding disorder. Disadvantages of nasotracheal intubation include the risk of bleeding in the posterior pharynx, risk of cranial placement in cases of basilar skull fracture, and high risk of infection.

Nasotracheal intubation is a blind insertion technique in which there is no direct visualization of the vocal cords and, as such, the risk of esophageal intubation is increased. Many sources recommend utilizing a laryngoscope and **Magill forceps** to visualize the glottis and facilitate passage of the endotracheal tube. But, if use of the laryngoscope and Magill forceps were to be tolerated by the patient an orotracheal intubation would be possible and preferred. In addition, you can aid the nasotracheal route by combining a digital intubation approach and using your fingers to guide the endotracheal tube into the glottis. Be careful about sticking your fingers into the patient's mouth, because if you elicit a gag reflex and the patient clamps down, you may get bitten.

Once nasotracheal intubation has been chosen as the means to obtain a patent airway, you will need to do a couple of things to make intubating easier on you and the patient. Choosing the right size endotracheal tube is very important. Make sure that the diameter of the endotracheal tube does not exceed the diameter of the patient's nares. As a rule of thumb, a endotracheal tube that is 0.5 mm smaller than one you would use if you were intubating orally is appropriate. The right nare is the larger of the two in most patients, and should be utilized first. If you meet resistance when inserting the tube, do not try to force the tube through the nare. Simply pull the tube out, and try again in the left nare.

It is helpful to use **Neo-Synephrine** or some other nasal decongestant spray, which will cause vasoconstriction in the nasopharynx. Vasoconstriction is a desirable effect that will help reduce the amount of bleeding, if any, caused by inserting the **endotracheal** tube. You will also need to lube the tip of the endotracheal tube with lidocaine jelly. This will help not only ease the insertion of the endotracheal tube, but will also numb the nasal tissue, making insertion of the tube more comfortable for conscious patients. If lidocaine jelly is not available, a lidocaine spray, or some other topical anesthetic spray, can be used to anesthetize the nasal and pharyngeal tissue. In addition, use a water-based lubricant to facilitate passage of the tube.

There are adjuncts that can help to facilitate a successful nasotracheal intubation. Two of these are the **Endotrol® endotracheal tube** (Figure 5.1) and the **Beck Airway Airflow Modulator (BAAM®)** (Figure 5.2). The Endotrol® endotracheal tube is a specialized endotracheal tube with a cord and ring attached to it. While inserting the endotracheal tube, pulling on the ring creates tension in the cord, bringing the tip of the tube more anterior to allow for easier insertion into the trachea. The BAAM® is a disposable device that is attached to the 15-mm endotracheal tube adapter and magnifies airway-airflow sounds of the patient's respirations by the means of a whistling noise. The whistling sound means that the tip of the endotracheal tube is close to the tracheal inlet. As you get closer to the tracheal inlet, the whistling noise gets louder. When you are closest to the vocal cords (when the whistling is the loudest), push the endotracheal tube down further past the vocal cords during inspiration. The whistling noise will get even louder, confirming that you are in the trachea.

If your agency does not provide the BAAM® for your use, then you can simply use your stethoscope. Take the entire bell off the end of your stethoscope, and place the stethoscope tube at the opening of the ETT. This allows you to listen for the sound of exhalations through your stethoscope. As the tip of the tube gets closer to the laryngeal inlet, the noise in your ears will get louder. Be cautious if you decide to just lean over the endotracheal tube and listen with your ear as opposed to using a stethoscope, as the patient may vomit on you if you elicit a gag reflex.

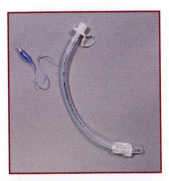

Figure 5.1

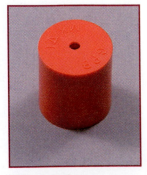

Figure 5.2

Just as with regular oral intubation, medications can be introduced down the tube when they are needed. The drugs that can be used down the endotracheal tube can be easily remembered by using either **LANE** (lidocaine, atropine, narcan, epinephrine) or **NAVEL** (narcan, atropine, water-based valium, vasopressin, epinephrine, lidocaine).

►EQUIPMENT

You will need the following equipment (Figure 5.3):

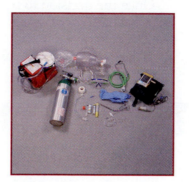

Figure 5.3

- ► Gloves
- ► Goggles
- ► Mask
- ► Oxygen tank with regulator
- ► Magill forceps
- ► End-tidal carbon dioxide ($ETCO_2$) detector
- ► Pulse oximeter, if available
- ► Suction equipment
- ► Endotracheal tube or Endotrol® endotracheal tube
- ► Stethoscope
- ► Bag-valve mask
- ► 10-cc syringe
- ► BAAM® (if available)
- ► Tape or commercial tube securing device
- ► Anesthetic spray (if available)
- ► Decongestant spray (if available)
- ► Lidocaine, KY jelly, or other lubricant
- ► Neo-Synephrine (if available)

ASSESSMENT

Assessment of a patient requiring nasotracheal intubation understandably centers on airway and breathing. If the patient is breathing but unable to protect the airway secondary to stroke, coma, oral trauma or an **areflexic** condition secondary to spinal trauma, nasotracheal intubation is indicated. Assessment findings that confirm the possible need for intubation include obvious respiratory distress; tachypnea; tachycardia; cool, pale, and diaphoretic skin; decreased SaO_2; use of accessory respiratory muscles; and positioning (such as tripoding). Ominous signs that indicate immediate need of airway control include bradypnea, cyanosis, altered mental status, unconsciousness, and any other indication of impending respiratory failure. Remember that while apnea is certainly an indication for endotracheal intubation, it is a contraindication for the nasal route, and would require an oral approach to intubation.

In addition to apnea, other contraindications for nasotracheal intubation include foreign body airway obstruction, bleeding disorders, severe facial trauma, and suspected basilar skull fracture. A patient who is breathing, as required for the nasotracheal route, cannot have a foreign body airway obstruction. However, a partial airway obstruction, as evidenced by stridorous breathing, may be present and should be ruled out. While the presence of serious facial trauma will be obvious upon examination, the signs of a basilar skull fracture can be subtle and need to be purposefully examined for signs of basilar skull fracture including Battle's sign (bruising just below and behind the ears), **periorbital ecchymosis**, and bleeding from the ear canal. While a bleeding disorder cannot usually be identified on physical exam, the patient can provide this information if you ask, or the patient may be wearing a MedicAlert bracelet stating such information. It is important to determine if the patient has a bleeding disorder because up to 70 percent of patients who are nasotracheal intubated have nasal bleeding secondary to this procedure.

Once the decision to perform nasotracheal intubation has been reached, a quick assessment of the nasal cavity should be performed to ensure that there are no obvious obstructions, deformities, or foreign bodies that would interfere with endotracheal tube insertion and passage.

PROCEDURE: Nasotracheal Intubation

1. Take infection control precautions.

   Rationale: Any airway management procedure is considered high risk or may result in possible exposure to infectious diseases since the possibility of spraying airway secretions exists. Gloves, goggles, and a mask are a must for airway management.

2. Ensure that basic life support airway management procedures continue while preparations are made for intubation, and place the patient on a pulse oximeter. Assist ventilations if necessary using a BVM device with 100 percent O_2. (Figure 5.4).

   Rationale: Administration of high-flow, high-concentration oxygen and assisting ventilations as needed are required to ensure the patient does not decompensate before the airway can be managed with intubation.

3. Select, assemble, and test the appropriate equipment.

   Rationale: There are many pieces of equipment required for proper airway management. Once engaged in the intubation procedure, failing to have a piece of equipment available and prepared could result in hypoxia for the patient.

PEDIATRIC NOTE:

The Broselow® Tape (see Chapter 25) can help to determine what size tube is needed for a pediatric patient. In the absence of a length-based resuscitation tape, some systems use a diameter of the child's little finger as a gross estimate of the outside diameter of the tube required.

4. Anesthetize and vasoconstrict the vessels in the nostrils and pharynx with spray anesthetic and Neo-Synephrine, respectively (Figure 5.5). Alternatively, topical anesthesia delivery can be accomplished with the use of lidocaine jelly.

GERIATRIC NOTE:

It is common for geriatric patients to have engorged nasal passages, making this step imperative to prevent nasopharynx bleeding that will necessitate suctioning.

Rationale: The anesthetic partially numbs the tissues, lessening patient discomfort, and topical vasoconstrictors such as Neo-Synephrine cause vasoconstriction, which reduces the size of the tissue and minimizes any potential bleeding from trauma caused by the nasotracheal tube.

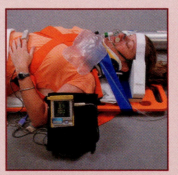
Figure 5.4

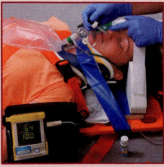
Figure 5.5

5. Lubricate the Endotrol® endotracheal tube with lidocaine or KY jelly (Figure 5.6).

Rationale: Lubricant will minimize potential abrasions or lacerations caused during the passing of the tube through the nasopharynx.

6. Attach BAAM® to the endotracheal tube if desired.

Rationale: The BAAM® is a listening device that assists the rescuer in knowing when the patient is inhaling and exhaling. The tube should only be inserted into the trachea when the patient is inhaling because that is when the vocal cords are open the widest. To do so when the cords are closed would result in severe airway damage.

7. Gently insert the Endotrol® endotracheal tube into the largest nare (usually the right) following the curvature of the nasopharynx. The BAAM® will whistle with the patient's respirations, and assist in identifying the location of the glottis; as the tip of the endotracheal tube moves closer to the glottis, the whistling sound will increase in intensity. The distal end of the Endotrol® endotracheal tube can be manipulated anteriorly by pulling on the ring, and laterally by twisting the tube to the right and left (Figure 5.7). Advance the tube into the trachea during patient inspiration (Figure 5.8).

Rationale: The tube needs to be inserted until the inflatable cuff is beyond the vocal cords, which is usually when the adapter is sitting flush with the nares. Otherwise, the cuff of the tube might be inflated above the cords in the hypopharynx, or within the glottis, causing a pressure ulcer on the cords themselves.

8. Inflate the distal cuff of the Endotrol® endotracheal tube using a 10-cc syringe (Figure 5.9).

Rationale: Inflation of the cuff prevents air leakage around the tube, which could potentially result in inadequate respirations, endotracheal tube displacement, or the aspiration of regurgitated stomach contents.

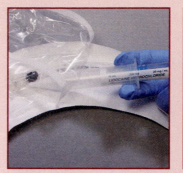
Figure 5.6

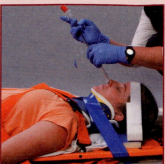
Figure 5.7

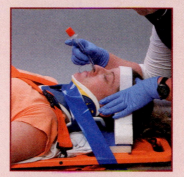
Figure 5.8

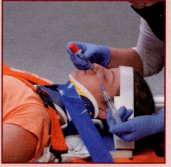
Figure 5.9

PEDIATRIC NOTE:

Remember that pediatric tracheal tubes are usually uncuffed; therefore, we will not require testing of the distal cuff during set-up for this procedure, or inflation after insertion into the trachea.

9. Remove the BAAM® and ventilate the patient using the bag-value mask while auscultating over the epigastrium for gurgling and observing for chest rise and fall. If you see no chest wall expansion with ventilation and hear sounds over the epigastrium you have intubated the esophagus. Stop ventilations and extubate the patient.

Rationale: Undetected esophageal intubation can be deadly for the patient. Reattempt ventilation after the patient has been reoxygenated with 100 percent oxygen for approximately 30 seconds. Assist ventilations as needed.

continued...

10. If there is an absence of sounds over the epigastrium and the chest wall expands with breaths, proceed with breath sound assessment over left and right anterior and axillary lung fields (Figure 5.10). Next observe for condensation in the ETT, and improving skin color.

    Rationale: Chest rise and fall, absent epigastrium sounds, lung field sounds, improving skin color, and condensation in the ETT are all primary assessment indicators of correct ET tube placement.

11. If lung sounds are auscultated on one side only, consider the need to adjust depth of tube placement by withdrawing the tube in small increments until it sits above the carina.

    Rationale: The patient is likely to be slightly hypoxic from the intubation procedure and will benefit from ventilation with high-flow oxygen. Observing for condensation in the tube, chest rise and fall, improvement of skin color, pulse oximetry and capnography are all methods of determining proper tube placement. Failure to use a combination of these methods could result in an inadvertent esophageal intubation remaining unidentified.

    Rationale: Chest rise and fall, absent epigastrium sounds, lung field sounds, improving skin color, and condensation in the ETT are all primary indicators of correct ET tube placement.

12. Confirm proper endotracheal tube placement with secondary assessment measures including $ETCO_2$ detectors, esophageal detector devices, auscultating lung sounds, condensation in the endotracheal tube, improving skin color, and increasing pulse oximetry. If lung sounds are auscultated on one side only, consider the need to adjust depth of tube placement by

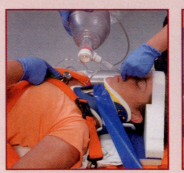
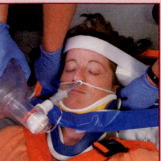

Figure 5.10   **Figure 5.11**

withdrawing the tube in small increments until it sits above the carina.

Rationale: The patient is likely to be slightly hypoxic from the intubation procedure and will benefit from ventilation with high-flow oxygen. Observing for condensation in the tube, chest rise and fall, improvement of skin color, pulse oximetry and capnography are all methods of determining proper tube placement. Failure to use a combination of these methods could result in an inadvertent esophageal intubation remaining unidentified.

13. Secure the endotracheal tube using tape or a commercial securing device (Figure 5.11).

    Rationale: Especially since nasotracheal intubation is only performed on breathing patients, there is a strong likelihood that the patient will move or accidentally dislodge the tube.

14. Continue assisting respirations with the bag-valve mask.

    Rationale: Now that the patient is intubated, breathing for the patient becomes the responsibility of rescuers.

ONGOING ASSESSMENT

Intubated patients must be reassessed regularly to ensure that the endotracheal tube remains in the trachea, and is not accidentally dislodged during patient movement. Confirmation of continued proper endotracheal tube placement is best accomplished through capnography. In addition, the observation of condensation inside the endotracheal tube, chest rise and fall, continued improvement of skin color, pulse oximetry, and auscultation of lung sounds with an absence of gastric sounds during ventilations are all indications that the endotracheal tube is still in place. During endotracheal intubation, direct visualization of the tube passing through the cords is also used to confirm tracheal placement. However, with nasotracheal intubation, visualization under direct laryngoscopy is often not possible since the patient is still breathing and usually has an intact gag reflex.

▶PROBLEM SOLVING

▶ If a BAAM® is unavailable to assist in identifying your patient's inhalations and exhalations, visualization of chest rise and fall, the assistance of a second rescuer for the latter, observation of condensation in the tube, or using the end of the stethoscope at the opening of the nasotracheal tube are all options for assisting in proper tube placement.

▶ No stylette is used during nasotracheal intubation, as it would render the endotracheal tube too rigid to travel through the curved nasopharynx; to do so would cause significant airway trauma.

▶ When performing a nasotracheal intubation, the patient will have some respiratory drive. Assisting ventilations with a bag-valve mask should be done in concert with the patient's own respirations. The bag should never be squeezed when the patient is exhaling.

▶ It is important to have the patient on a cardiac monitor to assist in the identification of dysrhythmias during nasotracheal intubation. Bradycardias are particularly common due to vagal stimulation. If the patient develops a lethal rhythm and apnea, orotracheal intubation should be performed instead.

▶CASE STUDY

You and your paramedic partner are dispatched to a local convalescent home for a possible stroke. Upon arrival at the facility, you are met by a member of the nursing staff who provides you with the patient's paperwork and a brief patient history as she walks with you to the patient's room. She states that a 73-year-old male in Room 4 has experienced an acute onset of left-sided paralysis immediately after returning to his room after lunch.

When you arrive at the patient's room, you note that the patient is sitting up in bed and leaning to his left. Your partner administers 100 percent oxygen via a nonrebreather mask at 15 lpm while you begin your interview. You note that he has **dysphonia**, **dysphagia**, and is experiencing a left-sided facial droop. The patient begins to regurgitate his lunch and seems to have a difficult time controlling his airway. Your partner removes the nonrebreather mask and suctions the patient's airway as you suggest performing a nasotracheal intubation. Your partner agrees, and you begin to set up the necessary equipment as your partner talks to the patient, advising him of the procedure you are going to perform.

As you attach the BAAM® to the 15-mm adapter of the Endotrol® endotracheal tube and apply lidocaine jelly to the distal tip, your partner sprays the patient's nasopharynx with Neo-Synephrine. You insert the endotracheal tube into the patient's right nare and advance it into the laryngopharynx and immediately hear the whistling of the BAAM® as the patient breathes. By twisting the Endotrol®

endotracheal tube and pulling on the ring, you are able to manipulate the distal end of the endotracheal tube to just above the glottis. As the patient takes a breath, you pass the tube through the glottic opening and into the trachea and hear a reassuring whistle from the BAAM® with each of the patient's breaths.

You inflate the cuff as your partner attaches an $ETCO_2$ detector and BVM to the endotracheal tube and begins to assist the patient's respirations. You immediately note a color change on the $ETCO_2$ detector, condensation in the endotracheal tube, bilateral chest rise and fall, increasing SaO_2, and bilateral and equal lung sounds on auscultation. Your capnometry reading is 38mmHg. You secure the endotracheal tube in place with tape, and then continue your physical exam prior to transporting the patient to the hospital without any further complications. ■

CHAPTER 6

Laryngoscopy with Magill Forceps

KEY TERMS

Aphagia

Direct laryngoscopy

Foreign body airway
    obstruction (FBAO)

Hypoxia

Laryngoscope

Laryngospasm

Magill forceps

OBJECTIVES

The student will be able to do the following:

▶ List the indications for performing laryngoscopy with Magill forceps
  on a patient (pp. 43–44).

▶ Describe the importance of properly performing laryngoscopy with
  Magill forceps on a patient (pp. 43–44).

▶ Describe the proper technique for performing laryngoscopy with
  Magill forceps on a patient (pp. 45–46).

▶ Demonstrate the ability to perform laryngoscopy with Magill forceps
  on a patient (pp. 45–46).

INTRODUCTION

A complete **foreign body airway obstruction (FBAO)**, the presence of
foreign material in the airway that completely blocks the airway and prevents ventilation, is always fatal if left untreated. Your patient will die unless the FBAO is removed, forced down a mainstem bronchus allowing
ventilation of the opposite lung, or totally bypassed with a surgical airway
located below the obstruction. **Direct laryngoscopy** and removal of the
obstruction with **Magill forceps** is the preferred method for removing a
foreign body airway obstruction that is unrelieved with BLS methods such
as abdominal thrusts, finger sweep, or chest thrusts. In addition to removing FBAOs, Magill forceps are used to assist nasotracheal intubation and
passing gastric tubes.

Direct laryngoscopy allows for visualization of the larynx, glottis, and
subglottic trachea and the identification of any obstruction located within
those areas. Magill forceps are anatomically shaped scissor-style clamps
with circular tips, designed to follow the contour of the oro- and hypopharynx when held in the right hand (**laryngoscope** in the left), and are

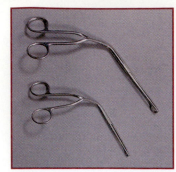

Figure 6.1

available in both pediatric and adult sizes (Figure 6.1). The clamps on older-style Magill forceps have serrated inner surfaces in order to give them an advantage in gripping objects. Newer, modified Magill forceps have smooth tips that reduce the risk of trauma to the mucous membranes, and also reduce the risk of perforating an endotracheal tube cuff when using Magills to assist in nasotracheal intubation.

Under direct laryngoscopy and with the Magill forceps held in the right hand, the forceps are inserted into the hypopharynx while closed, and opened only when you are prepared to grasp the obstruction. This helps prevent the forceps from obstructing your view of the obstruction, and reduces the risk of trauma from coming into contact with the pharyngeal anatomy.

In instances where a FBAO can be visualized below the vocal cords but not removed with the Magill forceps, an endotracheal tube with a stylet inserted can be used to push the obstruction further along the trachea and past the carina into the right mainstem bronchus. The endotracheal tube should then be removed and the patient's airway and breathing reassessed. Following failure to push the obstruction into the right mainstem, a surgical cricothyrotomy is indicated, or a needle cricothyrotomy can be performed if a surgical approach is not in your protocols.

The Magill forceps should be utilized in all instances of complete FBAO, and only in partial obstructions if the patient is unconscious. Suffice it to say that a conscious patient with a partial obstruction will not be compliant with the insertion of a laryngoscope into his or her airway. Due to the precarious nature of a partially obstructed airway, sedation or rapid sequence intubation (RSI) is not a recommended option; remember that a partial airway is better than none.

Most of your patients with FBAO will require some form of airway maintenance after removal of the obstruction. As such, it is a good idea to have a BVM attached to 100 percent oxygen, oro- and nasopharyngeal airways, a suction unit, and endotracheal intubation equipment prepared to address airway issues as they present themselves.

As a FBAO may be located at the vocal cords or even in the trachea, you should approach its removal much like you would an intubation to give yourself the best chance at visualizing the glottis (Chapters 1 and 3). Check your laryngoscope, use the same size blade that you would for endotracheal intubation, position the patient properly, and use proper intubation technique. FBAO technique and procedure is the same for adults and pediatric patients.

▶EQUIPMENT

You will need the following equipment (Figure 6.2):

▶ Gloves
▶ Goggles
▶ Mask
▶ Magill forceps
▶ Laryngoscope
▶ Suction unit
▶ Bag-valve mask
▶ Oxygen source
▶ Oropharyngeal airways
▶ Nasopharyngeal airways
▶ Nonrebreather mask

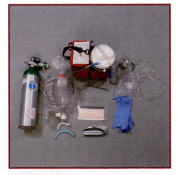

Figure 6.2

Place the patient in the supine position and determine her level of consciousness, as conscious patients cannot tolerate laryngoscopy. If the patient is conscious and she indicates, or you suspect, a FBAO, ask the patient if she can speak. If the patient can speak, she has a partial FBAO, not a complete, and no BLS or ALS FBAO removal maneuvers should be attempted. Signs of partial obstruction include stridor, difficulty breathing, and the presence of breath sounds. Signs of complete obstruction include the inability to speak, absent breath sounds, deep intercostal and supraclavicular retractions with inspiration attempts, worsening cyanosis, decreasing level of consciousness and eventual unconsciousness, and the inability to ventilate.

PROCEDURE: Laryngoscopy with Magill Forceps

1. Take infection control precautions.

   Rationale: Airway management puts rescuers at high risk of exposure to airway secretions. Gloves, goggles, and a mask are required for airway procedures.

2. Ensure that BLS FBAO removal techniques are being attempted while preparations are being made for direct laryngoscopy with Magill forceps.

   Rationale: BLS skills should always be attempted before invasive ALS procedures are utilized, as ALS procedures carry with them a higher risk of complication. BLS FBAO procedures include finger sweep, abdominal thrusts, and chest thrusts.

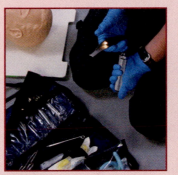

Figure 6.3

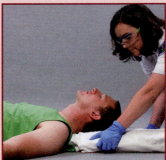

Figure 6.4

> ### PEDIATRIC NOTE:
>
> Abdominal thrusts (Heimlich maneuver) are performed the same way for both adults and children (> 1 year of age), with two exceptions. First, you may need to kneel behind the child to be at the proper height and you will want to squeeze the child victim more gently. For infants, (1 year of age), two fingers are used for chest thrusts on the mid-sternum.

functional bulb will prevent the rescuer from being able to visualize the vocal cords or the obstruction. Suction and BLS airway equipment should be readily available for post-FBAO removal airway issues.

4. Place the patient in a sniffing position and open his or her mouth (Figure 6.4).

   Rationale: The sniffing position puts the airway in the most accessible position. However, in the unusual event that trauma is associated with the choking, a neutral in-line position with manual cervical stabilization will be required.

3. Assemble and prepare your equipment by testing the light on the laryngoscope blade for tightness and brightness, and the suction for power (Figure 6.3).

   Rationale: A laryngoscope blade that is loose may dislodge into the patient's airway. A non-

> ### GERIATRIC NOTE:
>
> A patient with significant kyphosis may require padding under his or her head in order to achieve a neutral or sniffing position. Any resistance met by spinal abnormalities should not be forced.

continued...

5. Insert the laryngoscope blade and sweep the tongue to the left (Figure 6.5).

   Rationale: Moving the tongue out of the way will assist in visualizing the anatomy of the larynx and in locating the obstruction.

6. Advance the blade while visualizing the airway until the obstruction is seen (Figure 6.6). Suction as needed.

   Rationale: Fluid, secretions, or debris in the airway may prevent visualization of the obstruction itself.

7. Insert the Magill forceps with tips closed (Figure 6.7).

   Rationale: Open tips, especially serrated ones, can cause trauma to the oropharyngeal tissue.

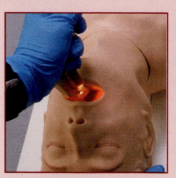
Figure 6.5

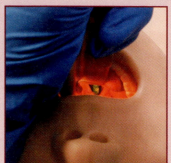
Figure 6.6

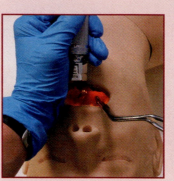
Figure 6.7

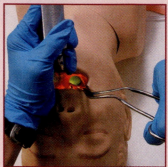
Figure 6.8

 PEDIATRIC NOTE:

Proper size equipment, including pediatric Magill forceps, is required for FBAO removal in a pediatric patient.

8. Open the forceps, grasp the foreign body tightly, and extract the obstructive material with a steady, firm pull (Figure 6.8).

   Rationale: Removal of the obstruction may require some force if it is deeply lodged into the airway, and pulling too quickly may cause you to lose grip of the obstruction.

GERIATRIC NOTE:

Food is the most common airway obstruction for adults. Geriatric patients are most likely to choke on food because they have decreased saliva production preventing the proper lubrication of food to facilitate swallowing. In addition, many stroke patients suffer from **aphagia,** or difficulty swallowing, which increases their risk of choking.

9. Remove the laryngoscope blade from the patient's airway (Figure 6.9).

   Rationale: Removing the laryngoscope allows you to assess the patient's airway and breathing.

10. Assess the patient's airway, breathing, and circulation.

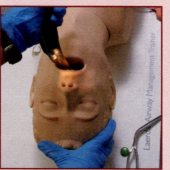
Figure 6.9

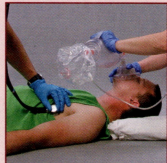
Figure 6.10

Rationale: Ensure that all of the obstructive material was removed, and that the patient has a patent airway, is breathing, and has a pulse.

11. Suction, provide supplemental oxygen, ventilate, or provide CPR as needed (Figure 6.10).

    Rationale: The patient was likely hypoxic for some time preceding the FBAO removal. Minimally, high-flow, high-concentration oxygen with a nonrebreather mask should be provided.

12. Dispose of the foreign body and airway equipment in an approved biohazard bag.

    Rationale: All airway equipment should be considered contaminated as it has likely come in contact with airway secretions.

Careful observation of the airway is required after removal of an airway obstruction. Often, the patient will begin breathing on his own, and have an adequate respiratory rate. Supplemental oxygen should be applied, even if the patient initially improves. The airway obstruction, as well as laryngoscopy, is traumatic and irritating to the oropharyngeal mucosa. Observe the patient to ensure that the insertion of the laryngoscope and Magill forceps did not cause swelling that later manifests in an occluded airway or **laryngospasm.** Should signs of airway edema or laryngospasm occur, such as hoarseness, stridor, or **hypoxia,** intubation should be considered.

▶ PROBLEM SOLVING

▶ The foreign body may be slippery, evading the grasp of the Magill forceps. Multiple attempts may be required to grasp the object and remove it.

▶ In some systems, if removal of the obstruction is impossible, pushing the obstruction further into the airway, past the carina, into the right or left mainstem bronchus is an approved technique. This procedure will cause an obstruction of either the right or left lung, but allows ventilation of the other. The foreign body can then later be removed from the lung with bronchoscopy.

▶ Laryngospasm is a dangerous complication of direct laryngoscopy. Should evidence of laryngospasm be noted, preparation should be made for immediate intubation before the laryngospasm results in a completely occluded airway.

▶ Be prepared to perform cricothyrotomy if attempts to clear the airway fail.

▶ CASE STUDY

You and your partner are dispatched to a local fast food restaurant for a patient who is not breathing. On the way to the call you think of the worst case scenario, cardiac arrest. When you get there, you see a young male in his 20s lying supine on the floor, cyanotic, with a bystander performing chest compressions. Witnesses say that the patient was having lunch and then suddenly stood up, clutching his throat. He did not make any noise, turned blue, and then passed out. The bystanders helped him onto the floor, and he did not strike his head.

You rule out the need for c-spine precautions, open the airway with a head tilt-chin lift, and look for the foreign object in the pharynx. Seeing nothing in the airway, you ask your partner to try to ventilate with the BVM. He states that he has a lot of resistance to bagging, so you reposition the patient's airway to no avail. You attempt a blind finger sweep, but do not remove or feel anything. You tell the bystander to resume chest compressions while you prepare your equipment for direct laryngoscopy with Magill forceps. You choose a Macintosh 3 laryngoscope blade, snap it into the handle, and ensure that the light is white, bright, and tight. You make sure the suction unit works and that it has a rigid-tip suction catheter attached. You grab the Magill forceps and position yourself at the patients head, insert the laryngoscope blade, sweep the tongue to the left, lift up the mandible, and see a large steak bolus lodged in the inferior hypopharynx, completely obscuring the glottic opening. You insert the Magill forceps, grasp the obstruction, and slowly but firmly pull the obstruction out of the airway.

The patient starts to cough and gag as you remove the laryngoscope, and you roll the patient onto his left side to help him keep his airway clear of secretions. The patient begins to cough more loudly and forcefully as he slowly regains color, and you provide him with blow-by oxygen as your partner listens to his lung sounds. ■

CHAPTER 7

Insertion of the Esophageal Tracheal Combitube®

KEY TERMS

Caustic substances

Distal cuff

Endotracheal intubation

Esophageal Tracheal
   Combitube® (ETC)

Extubation

Gag reflex

Gastric distension

Glottic opening

Hyperextend

Hypoxia

Jaw-lift maneuver

Pharyngeal cuff

Proximal

OBJECTIVES

The student will be able to do the following:

▶ List the indications for the placing of an Esophageal Tracheal
Combitube® in a patient (pp. 48–50).

▶ Describe the importance of properly placing an Esophageal Tracheal
Combitube® (pp. 48–50).

▶ List the contraindications for the placing of an Esophageal Tracheal
Combitube® (pp. 49–50).

▶ Describe the proper technique for inserting an Esophageal Tracheal
Combitube® (pp. 50–53).

▶ Demonstrate the ability to place an Esophageal Tracheal Combitube®
(pp. 50–53).

INTRODUCTION

The **Esophageal Tracheal Combitube®** is the primary backup airway in
most ALS systems. The device offers several major advantages. First, it uses
a "blind" insertion technique that does not require visualization of the trachea. Second, the Combitube® may prevent vomit from entering the trachea, thus protecting the airway. Third, the Combitube® allows for rapid
airway control independent of the patient's position. This is especially
helpful for trauma patients for whom limited movement of the cervical
spine is necessary.

    The Combitube® comes in two sizes, and as mentioned, requires no vi-
sualization of the glottic opening during the insertion process. It is a double lumen airway in which the two lumens are separated by a partition wall.
The Combitube® was developed to be placed in either the trachea or the
esophagus. The distal end of the Combitube® has a cuff that is used to seal

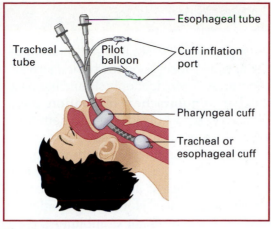

Figure 7.1

either the trachea or the esophagus, depending on where the airway is placed. The **proximal** end has a cuff used to seal the pharynx (Figure 7.1).

The #1 esophageal obturator tube is a little longer than the #2 tracheal tube and has a closed end. It delivers ventilations through small holes in the tubing between the **distal cuff** and the **pharyngeal cuff.** The perforations are just proximal to the **glottic opening**.

When the Combitube® is placed in the esophagus, the distal cuff will block the esophagus and the pharyngeal cuff will seal the mouth. During ventilations, the tube's sealed end prevents the ventilation from entering the esophagus and stomach. Ventilations flow out of the small holes into the pharynx and are diverted into the trachea and lungs. Esophageal placement occurs about 80 percent of the time with blind insertion.

The #2 tube has an open end similar to an endotracheal tube. If the Combitube® is placed into the trachea, the distal cuff and open distal end will ensure that ventilations are delivered directly into the trachea.

Use of the Combitube® is indicated in patients who are unconscious without a **gag reflex** for whom endotracheal intubation is required but attempts have proved unsuccessful. Contraindications to the use of the Combitube® include patients who are under 16 years of age, less than 5 feet tall, or greater than 7 feet tall. Ingestion of **caustic substances**, esophageal disease, and the presence of a gag reflex also exclude the use of the Combitube®.

▶EQUIPMENT

You will need the following equipment:

▶ Gloves
▶ Goggles
▶ Oxygen cylinder
▶ BVM and reservoir
▶ Suction equipment
▶ Combitube®
▶ Water-soluble lubricant
▶ Large 100-cc syringe
▶ Small 20-cc syringe
▶ Stethoscope

ASSESSMENT

Remember that use of the Combitube® is a BLS skill, and the assessment of a patient requiring use of the Combitube® focuses on the basics: airway, breathing, and circulation (ABCs). In addition, an ALS provider only should use a Combitube® after there has been a failure to intubate. **Endotracheal intubation**, not use of a Combitube®, is the ALS airway of choice. The most obvious assessment finding that should result in an immediate use of the Combitube® is apnea secondary to respiratory or cardiac arrest. This decision can become more involved in those patients who present in severe respiratory distress or extremis secondary to disease or trauma, as these patients will have some degree of consciousness and a gag reflex. Combitube® use is contraindicated in patients with a gag reflex. However, if a patient is in extremis, and BLS airway attempts and intubation attempts fail, Combitube® placement should be considered. In addition to having severe respiratory distress, patients in extremis who are in need of ETI will be tired, bradypneic, and have a decreased level of consciousness and an absent gag reflex; simply stated, these patients will be in impending respiratory arrest.

Unconsciousness in and of itself is not an absolute indication for Combitube® placement, but is when combined with a lack of a gag reflex and a risk of aspiration. As most patients in the prehospital environment can be assumed to have some gastric content, any patient without a gag reflex you encounter is a strong candidate for Combitube® use. Certainly, if your patient accepts an OPA and is receiving positive-pressure ventilations, a Combitube® is indicated unless you expect rapid improvement in the patient's condition, such as a hypoglycemic patient who is about to receive dextrose or a patient with a narcotic overdose who will be administered naloxone. If these patients are vomiting and the airway is uncontrollable, however, immediate insertion of the Combitube® may be required.

PROCEDURE: Insertion of the Esophageal Tracheal Combitube®

1. Apply BSI precautions.

   Rationale: Gloves and eye protection are required at a minimum, and a gown may be needed if large amounts of blood or fluid are present to prevent exposure to infectious diseases.

2. Ventilate the patient using a bag-mask device and 100 percent O_2, at a rate of 10-12 breaths/minute, (1 breath every 5-6 seconds), for at least 30 seconds, prior to intubation for perfusing patients, or 8-10 times per minute when CPR is in progress.

   Rationale: Oxygen saturation can drop precipitously during the intubation attempt causing the patient to become hypoxic during this procedure.

3. Place the patient in the supine position.

   Rationale: Maintaining proper anatomical alignment is important in this procedure. The Combitube® was developed to be placed in a patient only in the supine position but is sometimes used otherwise in trauma patients for whom limited movement of the cervical spine is necessary.

4. Position yourself at the patient's head.

   Rationale: This location is the best position for placement of the tube. If this position is not available, you may try from the side of the patient.

5. Rule out contraindications to insertion of the Combitube®. Confirm patient for proper age and size.

   Rationale: The Combitube® is contraindicated in patients who are less than 16 years, or less than 5 feet tall or over 7 feet tall.

6. Confirm that the patient does not have an active gag reflex.

Rationale: In a patient with an active gag reflex insertion of the tube can cause vomiting and potential aspiration.

7. Check the patient's past medical history to rule out esophageal disease.

    Rationale: Insertion of the Combitube® can cause rupture and bleeding of esophageal varices, a potentially life-threatening condition.

8. Confirm that the patient has not ingested any caustic substances.

    Rationale: Caustic substances may erode the esophageal lining causing bleeding or ulcerations.

9. If needed, suction any materials and/or fluids that might be obstructing the airway.

    Rationale: Aspiration of materials and/or fluid into the upper airway could happen if materials are not suctioned.

10. Assemble and check equipment, noting any air leaks in the cuffs (Figure 7.2).

    Rationale: Checking equipment now is essential to make sure that a problem does not occur during the insertion procedure. Later is not the time to find out that you have an equipment failure. Make sure that you maintain equipment in a clean environment. Foreign material on the Combitube® could cause an infection. Controversy surrounds whether the syringes should be attached to the Combitube® during insertion. Some individuals feel that it may make insertion more difficult with syringes attached.

11. Lubricate the distal end of the tube (Figure 7.3).

    Rationale: Lubrication of the tube allows for easier insertion and reduces the risk of trauma during insertion.

12. Keep the patient supine, with the head in a neutral, in-line position.

    Rationale: Maintaining the head in neutral alignment is important to maintain proper anatomical alignment.

13. Perform a **jaw-lift maneuver** (Figure 7.4).

    Rationale: This allows easy access to the oral cavity to insert the Combitube®. Be careful in performing this maneuver if the patient has experienced facial trauma or is even slightly conscious.

14. Place the Combitube® into the patient's mouth and gently insert the airway. It is important to note to yourself how long it is taking to perform

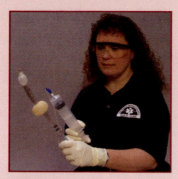
Figure 7.2

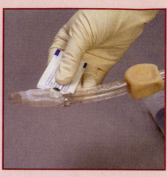
Figure 7.3

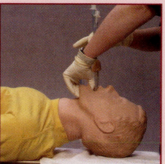
Figure 7.4

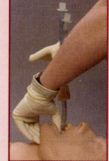
Figure 7.5

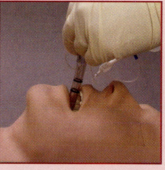
Figure 7.6

the Combitube® insertion. Do not attempt this procedure for longer than 30 seconds. If resistance is met, do not force the tube (Figure 7.5).

Rationale: Trauma to the upper airway could be caused by forceful insertion of the Combitube®. Patients can become hypoxic during this procedure.

15. Insert the Combitube® until the airway's black rings meet the level of the patient's teeth (Figure 7.6).

    Rationale: This is the point at which the Combitube® has been seated for proper positioning in the patient's airway.

continued...

16. Using the large syringe, inflate the pharyngeal cuff (blue) on tube #1 with 100 cc of air (Figure 7.7). (Use 85 cc of air for the smaller Combitube®.)

Rationale: The laryngeal cuff will rest at the hypopharynx. 100 cc of air will prevent air escape during ventilation.

17. Using the smaller syringe, inflate the distal cuff (white or clear) on tube #2 with 15 cc of air (Figure 7.8). (Use 12 cc of air for a smaller Combitube®.)

Rationale: The distal cuff will come to rest in the esophagus. 10-15 cc of air is enough to occlude the esophagus without causing damage to the esophageal tissue.

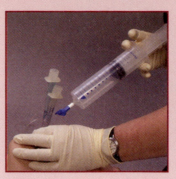
Figure 7.7

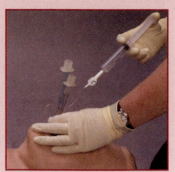
Figure 7.8

18. Attach the bag-mask ventilation device to tube #1 and slowly begin ventilations (Figure 7.9). Place a stethoscope over the patient's stomach and auscultate for gurgling sounds (Figure 7.10).

Rationale: Because you have blindly inserted the Combitube® into the airway, you will need to verify the tube location in either the esophagus or trachea.

19. If no sounds are heard over the patient's stomach, watch for chest rise, and auscultate the chest for breath sounds bilaterally. If the chest rises with each ventilation and you hear breath sounds, continue ventilations. Provide ventilations using the blue (pharyngeal lumen). Ventilate the patient using a bag ventilation device and 100 percent O_2 at a rate of 10-12 per minute if the patient has a perfusing rhythm and 8-10 breaths per minute if CPR is in progress. (It is permissible to do Step #18 and #19 in reverse order.)

Rationale: Signs of chest rise, breathe sounds, and NO stomach gurgling confirm that the Combitube® has been properly placed in the esophagus.

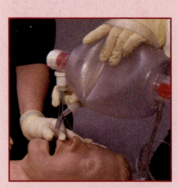
Figure 7.9

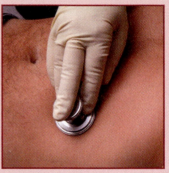
Figure 7.10

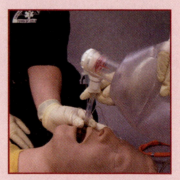
Figure 7.11

20. If gurgling sounds are present and you do not see chest rise and/or cannot hear breath sounds, your Combitube® was accidentally placed in the trachea. Immediately stop ventilations through tube #1 (blue lumen) once you are convinced the tube is located in the trachea.

Rationale: Additional ventilations into the stomach will increase the risk that the patient will vomit. Also prolonged ventilations into the stomach can cause **gastric distension**, resulting in pressure on the diaphragm and making ventilations of the lungs difficult.

21. Slowly begin ventilations through tube #2 (white or clear lumen) (Figure 7.11).

Rationale: Ventilation through tube #2 should ventilate the lungs directly.

22. Auscultate the stomach for gurgling sounds. Also look for chest rise, and auscultate the chest for bilateral breath sounds (Figure 7.12).

    Rationale: If gurgling sounds are heard during auscultation of the stomach, it could be an indicator that excessive air is entering the stomach and that the Combitube® is not placed correctly. If chest rise is not observed, and no lung sounds are heard during ventilation of either tube, continue to problem solve for possible misplacement of the Combitube® or ventilation through the wrong tube.

23. If there are NO epigastric sounds and if you see chest rise and/or hear breath sounds, continue ventilations (Figure 7.13).

    Rationale: When ventilating through tube #2, these signs of chest rise, breath sounds, and NO stomach gurgling confirm the location of the Combitube® in the trachea.

24. Although controversial, if at anytime you are confused or unsure of the location of the Combitube®, consider removing the tube, ventilating the patient for at least 30 seconds and trying again.

    Rationale: Being unsure of the placement of the Combitube® is not acceptable. Ventilating a

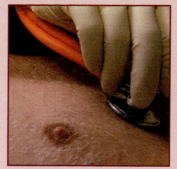

Figure 7.12

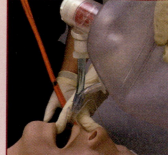

Figure 7.13

patient through the wrong tube could result in death or severe disability. You are better off starting over than being unsure of the Combitube's® location.

25. Insert an oropharyngeal airway (OPA) and continue to ventilate the patient.

    Rationale: The OPA will protect the tube in case the patient seizes or begins to awaken and bites down on the tube.

26. Document your findings.

    Rationale: It is extremely important to document your findings in order to have a history of facts and events that occurred at the scene.

ONGOING ASSESSMENT

Constantly monitor chest rise and watch for developing gastric distension. If ventilation of the lungs is accomplished, SaO_2 should begin to increase almost immediately. Monitor $ETCO_2$, if possible, and reassess frequently to assure continued ventilation. Monitor the pilot balloon on the end of each syringe tube. Each balloon should retain air pressure if the cuffs are adequately inflated. Re-evaluate lung sounds after every movement of the patient. Visualize the airway for materials and/or fluids.

▶ PROBLEM SOLVING

▶ If you meet resistance during the insertion process, do not force the tube. Forcing the tube could cause trauma to the upper or lower airways or to the esophagus.

▶ The major complication of the Combitube® is a failure to determine where the tube has been placed. You MUST assess the patient to make sure proper ventilations are being accomplished. If you are unsure of tube placement, remove the Combitube®, ventilate, and try again.

▶ Use care when inserting the Combitube® in patients who have sustained facial trauma.

- If you suspect cervical trauma, do not **hyperextend** the head during insertion of the Combitube®.

- **Hypoxia** can result if too much time is spent inserting the airway. If you suspect an extended time, remove the Combitube®, hyperventilate the patient, and try insertion again later.

- You must maintain adequate air pressure in both the pharyngeal and distal cuffs. Improper inflation can allow aspiration and/or cause air to leak from the tube. Monitor distal balloon pressure to ensure proper inflation.

- If the patient regains consciousness or demonstrates a gag reflex, remove the Combitube®. (Remember, vomiting almost always follows **extubation**.) For extubation, that is, to remove the Combitube®, take these steps:

  1. Apply BSI precautions.
  2. Have suction ready.
  3. Place the patient on his side.
  4. Deflate the pharyngeal cuff.
  5. Deflate the distal cuff.
  6. Remove the tube gently.
  7. Reassess the patient.
  8. Apply high-flow oxygen.

▶CASE STUDY

You are called as backup for a crew on scene with an intoxicated patient. When you arrive you find the original crew suctioning the patient. The patient is unresponsive, has vomited, and the crew is preparing to secure his airway. The patient remains unresponsive even with painful stimuli. During suctioning, you noticed that the patient did not have a gag reflex. Your partner elects to insert an oropharyngeal airway. The patient accepts the airway without difficulty.

You begin positive pressure ventilation, while your partner maintains cricoid pressure. The patient's level of responsiveness has not changed, so you decide to insert an advanced airway. Unfortunately, after two attempts, you are unable to successfully intubate the patient. Your partner suggests the Combitube®. You agree, and your partner begins to prepare the equipment while the patient is being hyperventilated. You take the Combitube® and insert it gently. Your partner assists you by inflating the cuffs. Your partner begins ventilating the patient through tube #1 while you listen over the epigastrium. You hear nothing and proceed to listen over the lungs. You confirm proper placement, and you begin to secure it. Your partner continues ventilating the patient as the remaining providers on scene package the patient for transport. Ventilations are continued through the Combitube® during transport, and the patient remains well oxygenated. Upon arrival at the emergency department, the patient care is transferred to the emergency staff. ■

CHAPTER 8

End-Tidal Carbon Dioxide Detection

KEY TERMS

Capnography

Capnometry

Colormetric

Hypercarbia

Hypocarbia

OBJECTIVES

The student will be able to do the following:

▶ List the indications for the application of a CO_2 detector (pp. 55–57).

▶ Describe the importance of proper application of a CO_2 detector (pp. 55–57).

▶ Describe the proper technique for the application and assessment of a CO_2 detector (pp. 58–59).

▶ Demonstrate the ability to apply a CO_2 detector properly (pp. 58–59).

INTRODUCTION

Intubation confirmation is a key component to patient survival. There are several standard primary confirmation techniques that rely on clinical assessment findings to confirm endotracheal tube (ETT) placement. Secondary confirmation techniques are not based on physical assessment findings and include esophageal detector devices, covered in Chapter 9, and devices that detect carbon dioxide (CO_2) exhaled through a properly placed ETT, known as end-tidal CO_2 (ETCO$_2$) detection devices.

The use of ETCO$_2$ detectors is recognized as the standard of care in the hospital setting by the American Society of Anesthesiologists. The National Association of Emergency Medical Services Physicians recommends the use of ETCO$_2$ detection devices as well as esophageal detection devices in the prehospital setting. As such, you should consider an ETCO$_2$ detection device, as well as an esophageal detection device, to be part of your intubation equipment, and it should be prepared prior to intubation like any other piece of equipment.

Determining the presence of ETCO$_2$ can be completed in one of two ways, either with a qualitative **colormetric** device that changes color in the presence of CO_2, or a quantitative device that gives a numerical readout or continuous capnographic waveform. The colormetric method of ETCO$_2$ detection is very quick, easy to use, economic, and is available in

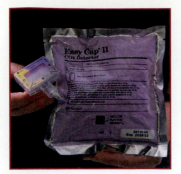

Figure 8.1

both pediatric and adult sizes (Figure 8.1). The devices are designed to be placed between a ventilation bag and the ETT via a 15-mm adapter. They come in several shapes, such as squares, circles, or even "T" adapters, and can also be found already built into the neck of a BVM device.

A piece of litmus paper inside the device changes color from purple (no CO_2) to yellow (CO_2 presence) with exhalation in a perfusing patient. The devices can be used to assist in the confirmation of ETT placement by any route, and to detect ranges of $ETCO_2$ that an intubated patient is exhaling, though this can be difficult, as it requires matching the color of the litmus paper to a color scale on the device or a separate chart. Normal $ETCO_2$ ranges with colormetric devices usually fall between 4.0–5.7 kPa, or 4.0–5.6 percent. Remember that the color scale on a colormetric device only provides an estimate of $ETCO_2$, and cannot accurately detect **hypocarbia** or **hypercarbia.**

Simply put, purple with no color change indicates that the ETT is not in the trachea, or that the ETT is in the trachea but the patient is in cardiac arrest. Color change from purple to yellow with each breath indicates tracheal placement of the ETT and that there is perfusion of the pulmonary vasculature (your patient has a pulse).

Colormetric $ETCO_2$ devices have some limitations. In cardiac arrest, $ETCO_2$ may be undetectable due to poor profusion. Even if the tube is properly placed in the trachea, CO_2 transport to, and elimination from, the lungs is significantly decreased. But the provider should keep in mind that, with proper CPR, it is possible to have slight color change if sufficient pulmonary blood flow is achieved. The $ETCO_2$ detector should be placed on patients in cardiac arrest, as it will respond immediately to the increase in CO_2 elimination should your patient regain pulses; in fact, color change on an $ETCO_2$ detector may be your first indication that a spontaneous return of circulation is present.

Colormetric $ETCO_2$ detectors cannot ensure that an ETT is inserted to a proper depth, requiring that you confirm tracheal placement, and not mainstem placement, with auscultation of lung sounds.

In addition, the $ETCO_2$ detector may react to CO_2 in the esophagus, resulting in a false positive (ETT is thought to be in the trachea when it is actually in the esophagus) and possible unrecognized esophageal intubation. Situations such as carbonated beverages in the stomach, and swallowed or forced air from the patient's hypopharynx (originally from the lungs, containing CO_2), delivered to the esophagus have been reported to have resulted in such false positives. In such cases, the persons involved reported noting a "tan" color on the $ETCO_2$ detector, or a color change between purple and yellow, a result of the small amounts of CO_2 present.

To prevent such events from taking place, a manufacturer recommends that six breaths be administered before checking for color change on the device, thus "washing out" any esophageal CO_2 that may be present. The result would be an unchanging purple color on the device, indicating either esophageal placement or a cardiac arrest situation. This actually works to your advantage, allowing you to auscultate for breath and epigastric sounds with the first six breaths prior to assessing for color change.

Colormetric $ETCO_2$ detectors should not be used during mouth-to-tube, or mouth-to-mouth, ventilations, nor around certain chemicals, such as anesthetics, or excessive humidified areas, such as nebulizers or heated humidifiers. In addition, these devices should not come in contact with gastric contents, mucus, or epinephrine. All of these situations can cause the paper to give a false, or wrong, $ETCO_2$ reading that does not change with the respiratory cycle.

This type of device will be difficult to analyze for those individuals with blue-yellow color blindness.

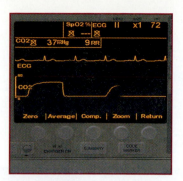

Figure 8.2

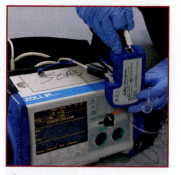

Figure 8.3

Quantitative end-tidal CO_2 detector monitors are considered by many to be the best method for secondary confirmation of the ET tube. The capnographic devices (Figure 8.2) give a continuous waveform display of the level of CO2 present throughout the ventilation cycle. The capnometric devices can be hand-held and give a single numeric value of CO_2 concentration at the time the measurement is taken. Many portable monitors and ventilator machines now come standard with capnographic or capnometric capabilities (Figure 8.3). Instead of reading a piece of paper, and guessing the range of $ETCO_2$, now a graphic waveform can be seen (referred to as **capnography**), or the actual mmHg or torr can be determined (called **capnometry**). A normal capnogram is the best evidence that the ETT is in the correct place. Reading how the waveforms present shows validation of $ETCO_2$ value, visual assessment of patent airway, verification of proper tube placement, and assessment of ventilator and breathing circuit integrity. It is a great indicator of the effectiveness of CPR, and can give a rapid assessment of cardiopulmonary status.

It is fairly easy to read the capnometry display, a digital number somewhere on the screen that is displayed in mmHg or torr. Normal $ETCO_2$, the range of someone who has good metabolic processes and is efficiently exchanging CO_2 with the outside environment, is around 35–45 mmHg.

Just like with the colormetric device, the plug for the capnograph and capnometer goes in-line to the patient's respirations, between the ETT and the BVM or ventilator tube. An infrared beam is passed through a sample of exhaled gas containing CO_2, and the ratio of light absorbed to light transmitted is examined to determine the concentration of CO_2. The advantages of using this technology are that it is fast acting, will not give false reading with emesis or medications, and it can also be utilized in non-intubated patients by using a commercially available, modified nasal cannula.

►EQUIPMENT

You will need the following equipment (Figure 8.4):

► Gloves
► Goggles
► Stethoscope
► Bag-valve mask
► Oxygen source
► Intubated patient
► CO_2 detection device

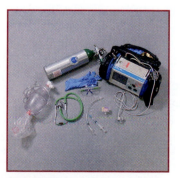

Figure 8.4

▶ASSESSMENT

Every intubated patient should have the benefit of ETCO$_2$ monitoring as it is the only device that will give immediate feedback if the tube becomes dislodged or the patient regains pulses.

PROCEDURE: End-Tidal Carbon Dioxide Detection

1. Take infection control precautions.

   Rationale: Gloves and goggles are a must when working around the airway since respiratory particles can contain infectious microorganisms.

2. Check the colormetric device for the integrity of the package, expiration date, and purple color, and assemble the capnometry device.

   Rationale: If the package is damaged or equipment is defective, an inaccurate or false capnometry reading may be obtained.

3. Perform intubation, auscultate lung sounds and epigastrium, and then connect the colormetric device (Figure 8.5) or capnometer (Figure 8.6) between the BVM and the end of the ETT.

   Rationale: The device detects or measures expired carbon dioxide which will exit the respiratory tract through the end of the ETT.

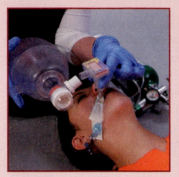
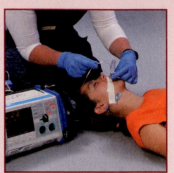

Figure 8.5   **Figure 8.6**

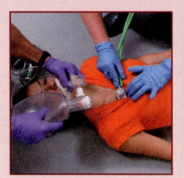
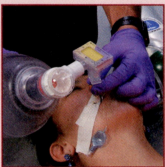

Figure 8.7   **Figure 8.8**

PEDIATRIC NOTE:

An adult colormetric device should not be used on patients under 15 kg. A special pediatric sized CO$_2$ detector should be used for accurate readings.

4. Perform, or instruct your assistant to perform, BVM ventilations for at least six breaths before observing for color change during expirations or reading the capnometry measurement on the monitor. Use this opportunity to assess breath sounds (Figure 8.7).

   Rationale: Six breaths provide enough air exchange to remove any CO$_2$ from the esophagus in the case of esophageal intubation, allowing for identification of esophageal placement of the

ETT. Auscultating breath sounds is a primary method of confirming proper tube placement and depth.

5. Determine colormetric device color or capnometer reading and action required.

   Rationale: If the colormetric device changes from purple to yellow with each exhalation, leave the tube and detector in place (Figure 8.8). If the colormetric device turns tan with each exhalation, give six more breaths and then reassess tube placement and detector for subsequent color change (Figure 8.9). If the colormetric device remains purple with exhalation, consider extubation (Figure 8.10).

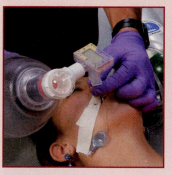

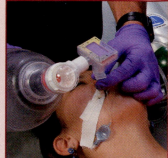

Figure 8.9   **Figure 8.10**

> ### GERIATRIC NOTE:
>
> Elderly patients are likely to be apneic as a result of cardiac arrest: Remember that the device may remain purple on a non-perfusing patient even if the tube is properly placed in the trachea.

ONGOING ASSESSMENT

Since the capnometer will be used on an intubated patient who is likely in respiratory arrest, this patient is critical. Reassessment of a full set of vital signs is indicated every 5 minutes for critical patients. However, reassessment of specific elements of the airway and breathing status are also important when caring for an intubated patient (Figure 8.11).

The capnometer can actually aid in assessment of the airway and breathing since a visual cue is given regarding the status of respiration. The numerical reading on the capnometer or the color on a colormetric device can assist with ongoing tube placement verification. When a change is noted on either device, such as the numerical value dropping significantly or the color changing from yellow to purple, the rescuer is cued to begin reassessment of tube placement, equipment function, breathing status, respiratory values, and so on.

The intubated patient should have frequent reassessment of the patency of the airway, tube cuff pressure, BVM function, chest rise, condensation in the tube on exhalation, lung sounds, and the absence of epigastric sounds. Any patient movement on scene, during transport, at arrival at the ED, during compressions, or during medication administration can all result in a dislodged tube. The colormetric device can assist in detection of a dislodged tube (sudden cessation of color change) for immediate correction by the rescuer (Figure 8.12).

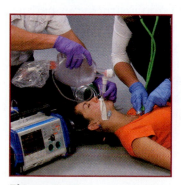

Figure 8.11

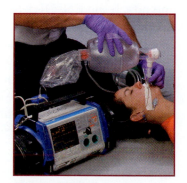

Figure 8.12

▶ PROBLEM SOLVING

▶ The colormetric device relies on a piece of litmus paper within the device to determine the presence of carbon dioxide and the resultant color change. If the paper gets wet, the device will fail to change color. Dispose of the device if you suspect it could have become wet with respiratory secretions, blood, or vomit.

▶ When using the colormetric device, it is recommended that it be removed after the initial determination of tube placement. Prolonged use will cause the device to get wet with condensation, causing inaccurate readings.

▶ Colormetric devices have an expiration date on the package, much like medications and IV fluid. If the package is expired, results will be unreliable. Dispose of the device and use one that has not yet exceeded the expiration date.

▶ Sometimes the colormetric device will remain purple when used on non-perfusing patients such as those in cardiac arrest because not enough blood is returned to the heart and lungs to exhale a measurable amount of carbon dioxide. If this occurs, document the finding and rely on other signs to confirm tube placement such as visualization of the vocal cords, chest rise, lung sounds, or condensation in the tube.

▶ When using capnographic waveform the sudden absence of a waveform and a drop in the numerical capnometry reading to zero or single digits can be your most reliable indicator of a displaced ET tube. Immediately reassess as your patient will likely need to be extubated.

▶ CASE STUDY

You and your partner respond to the home of a 75-year-old female where CPR is in progress. When you reach the patient, you notice that the patient's sons are performing effective CPR, and you ask everyone to step back. You check for breathing and a pulse, but nothing is palpable or noted. You use the paddles of your defibrillator to perform a quick look and see that the patient is in PEA. You delegate compressions back to the patient's son, and ask your partner to insert an OPA and provide ventilations with a BVM and high-flow high-concentration oxygen while you prepare your ET equipment.

Along with the laryngoscope, endotracheal tube, and esophageal detector device, you ready a colormetric $ETCO_2$ detector, ensuring that it has not expired, the packaging is intact, and that the litmus paper is purple when you remove it from the packaging. CPR and ventilations are stopped while you successfully intubate your patient and attach the $ETCO_2$ detector between the BVM and ETT. You instruct your partner to begin BVM ventilations as you auscultate the epigastric area and lung fields. He reports that there is no color change on the $ETCO_2$ detector, but you reply that the patient is in cardiac arrest, and you saw the ETT go through the cords, see chest rise and fall, hear equal lung sounds bilaterally, and hear nothing over the epigastric region; therefore, you are sure that the ETT is in the trachea. You secure the ETT, reassess equal and bilateral lung sounds, and follow local protocols for PEA. ■

CHAPTER 9

Use of the Esophageal Detector Device

KEY TERMS

End-tidal carbon dioxide detectors (ETCO₂)

Esophageal detector devices (EDDs)

Esophageal intubation

Esophageal intubation detectors (EIDs)

OBJECTIVES

The student will be able to do the following:

▶ List the indications for the application of an esophageal detector device to a patient (pp. 61–62).

▶ Describe the importance of proper application of an esophageal detector device (pp. 61–62).

▶ Describe the proper technique utilized in the application and use of an esophageal detector device (pp. 63–64).

▶ Demonstrate the ability to properly apply and use an esophageal detector device (pp. 63–64).

INTRODUCTION

Early and irrefutable confirmation of endotracheal tube (ETT) placement is crucial in the survival of any intubated patient. **End-tidal carbon dioxide detectors (ETCO₂)**, capnography, and direct visualization of the tube through the vocal cords remain the gold standards for confirmation of endotracheal tube (ETT) placement in the field. However, **esophageal detector devices (EDDs)**, also called **esophageal intubation detectors (EIDs),** have grown to become a favorite in the prehospital setting. In certain cases where insufficient volumes of CO_2 are produced, such as in cases of cardiac arrest or severe bronchospasm, $ETCO_2$ devices have been proven to be unreliable indicators of endotracheal placement of the tube, making EDDs a good alternative or supplemental means of ETT placement verification. There are two basic forms of the EDD: the syringe device and the self-inflating bulb device.

Both of these devices work under the same principle; they create negative pressure. The anatomical characteristics of the trachea and esophagus create different situations when negative pressure is applied with the EDD. If the device is applied to the proximal end of an ETT that has been placed in the trachea and negative pressure is applied, the cartilaginous tracheal rings will support the walls of the trachea, preventing collapse around the distal end of the ETT. As a result, a depressed, self-inflating bulb device placed on the proximal end of an ETT placed in the trachea will reinflate within 4 seconds. If you use a syringe-type device, you will be able to easily pull back on the syringe plunger and aspirate air from the trachea.

If the EDD is applied to the proximal end of an ETT that has been placed in the esophagus, the unsupported, smooth muscle walls of the esophagus will collapse around the distal end of the ETT when negative pressure is created. This results in delayed or no reinflation of the self-inflating bulb device, or resistance felt when the plunger of a syringe device is pulled back.

With both of these devices, many systems teach providers not to ventilate the patient through the ETT prior to application and use of the EDD, as it is believed that air introduced into the esophagus may result in esophageal distension and a false positive result (the ETT is in the esophagus but the bulb inflates) when there is no resistance to reinflation of the bulb or withdrawal of the syringe.

There are several advantages to using either of these devices. They are both easy to use, reliable, can be used in a noisy environment, do not require electricity, do not need to be calibrated nor require you to guess what color things might be, and they give you fast, immediate results. In addition, these devices are portable and disposable. The self-inflating bulb device has nearly 100 percent specificity and sensitivity for detecting **esophageal intubation** in adults, but false negatives and false positives can and do occur. Studies have shown that the self-inflating bulb device is more sensitive to esophageal placement than is the syringe device.

The syringe-type EDD is a 60–100 cc syringe with a 15-mm ETT adapter attached to the needle hub adapter on the distal end. The plunger end of the syringe contains a ring that helps draw back, or aspirate the plunger. It is important to work the plunger back and forth inside the barrel of the syringe to ensure that the plunger is not adhered to the barrel surface, a common occurrence as a result of the manufacturing process.

Before ventilations are performed, and with the plunger compressed all the way down, place the ET adapter onto the end of the inserted ETT. Once attached, withdraw the plunger from the syringe barrel by pulling up on the plunger ring, as you would withdraw medication from a vial. If aspiration is easy and no resistance is felt, then you are in the trachea. If aspiration is difficult or no air can be aspirated, then you are in the esophagus. If you have successful aspiration, hold onto the ETT, take off the EDD, and begin to ventilate your patient, confirming endotracheal (ET) placement and proper depth by auscultation of bilateral lung sounds. If you are unsuccessful with aspiration, extubate your patient, provide ventilations with a BVM and 100 percent oxygen for at least 30 seconds, then reattempt intubation.

The bulb-type EDD works in much the same way, and also needs to be used before ventilations are attempted to avoid a possible false positive result. The bulb-type EDD is round and has a 15-mm ETT adapter. Some manufacturers make this device so that it glows in the dark. To use, compress the bulb in your hand, attach it via the 15-mm ETT adapter to the proximal end of an inserted ETT, then release the bulb. A negative pressure is created at the end of the ETT, and rapid (< 4 seconds) reinflation of the bulb indicates tracheal placement of the ETT. Esophageal placement of the ETT is indicated if the bulb remains compressed or returns to the normal shape slowly.

▶EQUIPMENT

(Figure 9.1):

▶ Gloves
▶ Goggles
▶ Intubated patient
▶ Esophageal detector device

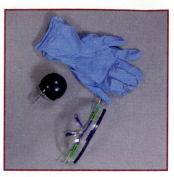

Figure 9.1

ASSESSMENT

There is no proper assessment, per se, for the application and use of an EDD, other than that there must be an ETT in place. Rather, you should remember that the device should be utilized whenever ET intubation is performed. Refer to Chapter 1 for the assessment of the patient requiring intubation.

 PROCEDURE: Use of the Esophageal Detector Device

1. Take infection control precautions.
   Rationale: Use of the EDD will occur during management of the airway, which puts the rescuer at risk for exposure to potentially infectious respiratory secretions.

2. Prepare EDD by either testing the bulb for pliability (Figure 9.2) or working the plunger within the barrel of the syringe.
   Rationale: Confirming that the equipment is in proper working order will help prevent a false reading or difficulty with the procedure.

3. If the patient is being ventilated by bag-valve mask, order ventilations to stop and remove the BVM from the end of the endotracheal tube (Figure 9.3).
   Rationale: The EDD must be placed on or in the end of the ET tube.

4. Attach the EDD to the end of the ETT (Figure 9.4).
   Rationale: The EDD will withdraw air from within the trachea or bronchi through the ETT if it is properly placed in the trachea.

5. Test for ETT placement in the trachea by either squeezing the bulb (Figure 9.5) or pulling back on the plunger of the syringe.

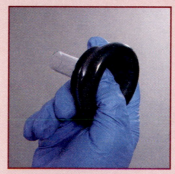

Figure 9.2

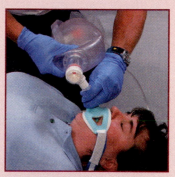

Figure 9.3

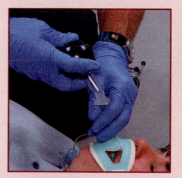

Figure 9.4

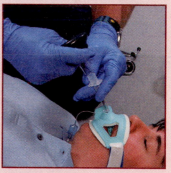

Figure 9.5

continued...

Rationale: If ETT is properly placed in the trachea, the bulb will reinflate (Figure 9.6). If using the syringe, it should be possible to aspirate air into the syringe. If the bulb remains deflated (Figure 9.7) or it is impossible to aspirate air into the syringe, it means that the flexible tissue of the esophagus has closed around the end of an improperly placed ETT.

> **PEDIATRIC NOTE:**
>
> Since the trachea of an infant or child is not yet closed into cartilaginous rings, but rather open on one side, EDDs should not be used on pediatric patients weighing less than 20 kg as it is possible to collapse the trachea around the tube, causing a false reading.

6. Observe results of the esophageal detection and take appropriate action. If the bulb inflated or the syringe aspirated air, resume ventilations (Figure 9.8). If it was determined that the tube was placed in the esophagus, begin extubation (Figure 9.9).

   Rationale: Ventilations, whether provided through the ETT or with a BVM and face mask, should be initiated as soon as possible to prevent hypoxemia.

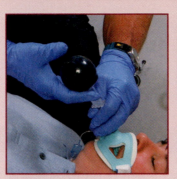

Figure 9.6

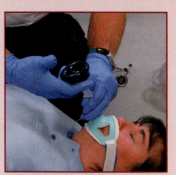

Figure 9.7

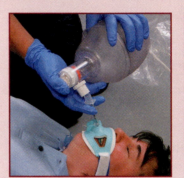

Figure 9.8

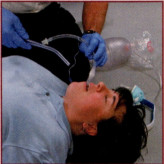

Figure 9.9

ONGOING ASSESSMENT

Once the results of the initial esophageal detection are received, it is rarely necessary to repeat the procedure. However, the principle of the procedure remains the same whether used during an initial intubation or for confirmation of tube placement after patient movement. If it is ever suspected that the tube may have been dislodged, or a finding of concern occurs, such as poor chest rise, absent or decreased lung sounds, difficulty ventilating, decreasing SaO_2, changes in skin color, or tachycardia, it is appropriate to disconnect the BVM momentarily to repeat the EDD procedure and confirm continued tube placement. If during reassessment the bulb fails to reinflate or it is no longer possible to aspirate the syringe, it is probable that the tube has been dislodged and immediate extubation should be considered.

▶ PROBLEM SOLVING

▶ If, by using the EDD during transport, it is determined that the tube was initially properly placed but has become dislodged, extubate the patient and provide ventilations with a BVM and 100 percent oxygen. Should your system require contact with medical control prior to extubation, do it expeditiously so as to extubate and provide BVM ventilations as quickly as possible.

▶ Since most EDDs are made of plastic, heat and cold may affect the function of the device. Heat can degrade or even melt plastic, and cold, dry air can cause the plastic to crack. Attempt to keep all airway equipment at room temperature and not exposed to severe temperatures in outside cabinets.

▶CASE STUDY

You and your partner are dispatched to an MVC on a busy interstate highway. Upon arrival you notice the driver is pinned in the car and in respiratory arrest. You get out the BVM, hook it up to high-flow, high-concentration oxygen, and begin to ventilate the patient while your partner holds the c-spine. You note that the tongue is acting as an airway obstruction, making ventilation difficult, so you place an OPA and continue to ventilate. The lieutenant of the rescue company tells you that it will take another 7 minutes to extricate the patient from the car. You have a firefighter take over ventilations while you prepare your intubation equipment. While facing the patient from the hood of the car, you perform a face-to-face intubation.

The environment is very noisy due to the use of extrication tools, so you know that you will be unable to auscultate lung sounds reliably, and it is difficult to see past the upper torso of the patient due to the dashboard that is compressing her chest. Before ventilating the patient, you attach your syringe-type EDD and are able to aspirate 50 ccs of air without any difficulty. You immediately take off the EDD, attach the BVM, and begin to ventilate your patient. You visualize condensation in the ETT and ventilate until the patient is freed from the car. ■

CHAPTER 10

Pulse Oximetry

KEY TERMS

Acetone wipes

Hemoglobin

Hypoxia

Oxygen saturation
  percentages

Pulse oximeter

OBJECTIVES

The student will be able to do the following:

▶ List the indications for the application of a pulse oximeter on a patient (pp. 66–67).

▶ Discuss the importance of proper application of a pulse oximeter (pp. 66–67).

▶ Describe the proper technique used for applying a pulse oximeter (pp. 67–68).

▶ Demonstrate the ability to apply a pulse oximeter (pp. 67–68).

INTRODUCTION

A **pulse oximeter** is a photoelectric device that measures the level of oxygen circulating in a patient's blood vessels. It consists of a portable monitor and a sensing probe.

An oximeter's sensor is most commonly clipped onto a fingertip, toe, earlobe, or, in the case of an infant, the distal foot. Once activated, the device sends different colors of light into the tissue and measures the amount of light that returns. It records the results as the **hemoglobin** saturation percentage and, in the case of oxygen, may be recorded as SpO_2. The measurements are affected by the percentage of any molecule bound to hemoglobin. In most cases, this is a measure of oxygen.

Normally, the SpO_2 is between 95 to 100 percent. **Oxygen saturation percentages** below 95 percent may represent varying levels of **hypoxia**. Be aware, however, that some patients may present normally with a SpO_2 of less than 95 percent. A good example would be a chronic obstructive pulmonary disease (COPD) patient.

Instead of relying solely on the pulse oximeter, incorporate it into your overall clinical assessment. Any patient who complains of respiratory difficulty or who exhibits an altered mental status should be assessed with a pulse oximeter, and some systems advocate use on every patient. This is a noninvasive device without any notable complications except when it distracts you from other indications of the patient's condition. Treat the patient—not the device.

Often called the "fifth vital sign," pulse oximetry should be part of every vital sign determination. As such, it is indicated any time you perform an assessment and is especially useful in the assessment of any patient with the potential for respiratory compromise instability. Pulse oximetry does not take the place of any component of the primary exam, however. Conditions that can affect the accuracy of the pulse oximeter include anemia, carbon monoxide poisoning, or any condition that causes poor peripheral perfusion.

In addition to its value as a vital sign, pulse oximetry is useful in helping to evaluate the effectiveness of treatments, such as oxygen therapy, ventilation, and medication administration, and in identifying deteriorating patients.

Each device comes with a manual on how to operate that particular device. It is essential for you to become familiar with the workings of that particular device. These procedures will make you familiar with the generic procedures of a pulse oximeter.

►EQUIPMENT

You will need the following equipment:

► Pulse oximeter
► Various sizes of probes (adult, pediatric, infant)
► Extra batteries
► **Acetone wipes** (to remove fingernail polish)

ASSESSMENT

As previously stated, pulse oximetry can be considered the "fifth vital sign," and as such should be utilized any time you perform a patient assessment.

Of particular concern should be those patients who present with respiratory distress. Any signs or symptoms of respiratory distress, including dyspnea; tachypnea; bradypnea; tachycardia; increased work of breathing; cyanotic or pale, cold, and diaphoretic skin; or adventitious lung sounds, warrant a determination of SpO_2.

PROCEDURE: Pulse Oximetry

1. Apply BSI precautions.

   Rationale: Gloves and eye protection are required at a minimum, and a gown may be needed if large amounts of blood or fluid are present to prevent exposure to infectious diseases.

2. Connect the sensor lead to the monitor and clip the sensor probe to the patient's fingertip on a noninjured extremity (Figure 10.1). Determine the patient's pulse rate.

   Rationale: Although other types of probes are available, finger probes seem to be the most comfortable and nonintrusive to patients. In most cases the finger probe is a reusable device.

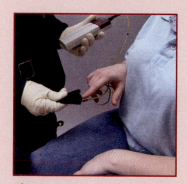

Figure 10.1

continued...

An injured extremity may give a false or no reading.

3. Turn on the pulse oximeter.

   Rationale: The pulse oximeter will not work if the power is not on.

4. Observe for the SpO_2 and heart rate. Make sure the heart rate displayed on the monitor screen is the same as the patient's pulse rate (Figure 10.2).

   Rationale: It may take a few seconds for the device to get a reading. The patient's pulse and the heart rate on the pulse oximeter should be the same. If they are not, consider moving the probe to another finger.

5. Some pulse oximeters may display a pulsatile waveform, which should correspond with the patient's pulse rate.

   Rationale: You can use the wave form to confirm heart rate, but a manual pulse rate should always be taken as the machine will only detect good blood flow. A patient with compromised circulation, such as hypovolemia, may have an inaccurate heart rate reading on the pulse oximeter.

6. Once you get an accurate reading, check the oximeter reading every 5 minutes, or if the patient

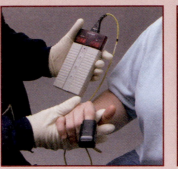 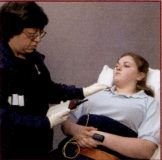

Figure 10.2   **Figure 10.3**

suddenly becomes more short of breath or shows signs of hypoxia. A convenient time to do this is when you check the patient's vital signs (Figure 10.3).

Rationale: It is important that, if you have placed a pulse oximeter on the patient, you constantly monitor the readings. Changes in oximetry readings should be documented. Some oximeter devices have alarms that can be set if the pulse oximetry reading drops below a preset level.

7. Document the SpO_2 measurement.

   Rationale: It is extremely important to document your findings in order to have a history of facts and events that occurred at the scene.

ONGOING ASSESSMENT

Constantly check to make sure that the sensor probe is still attached to the patient. Movement of the patient, either voluntarily or involuntarily, may dislodge the probe. You might turn on the pulse oximeter's alarm, which will alert you if the probe becomes dislodged. Also, note that some models turn themselves off after a period of inactivity.

▶PROBLEM SOLVING

▶ If you think the sensor probe may become easily dislodged, consider securing it in place with tape.

▶ If you're unable to obtain a reading or if you get poor waveforms or a "trouble" indicator, consider repositioning the sensor probe or moving it to an alternate site. Check to ensure that the batteries are functioning; if they are not, change the batteries.

▶ In patients with poor peripheral perfusion, the earlobe may give more accurate reading as it is more central than the fingers or toes.

- Some fingernail polish and fingernail embellishments, such as acrylic nails and decals or stones placed on the nail, can interfere with pulse oximeter measurements. If present, acetone wipes should be used before attaching the sensor probe. Acetone wipes should be stored with the pulse oximeter.
- Regardless of the pulse oximeter reading, watch for and treat signs of hypoxia such as restlessness, anxiety, confusion, or change in skin color.

►CASE STUDY

You and your partner have been called to the home of a 30-year-old male who is having difficulty breathing. When you arrive, you find him sitting in a chair in the kitchen, wheezing loudly. The patient states that he has a history of asthma, and his difficulty breathing started approximately a half hour before calling for help. He states that he used his inhaler once with no relief.

On your initial assessment, his skin is warm and dry and he has a strong pulse. Your partner obtains baseline vital signs, and reports that the patient is breathing at 32 times per minute, has a heart rate of 96, and has a blood pressure of 132/76. You place the pulse oximeter on the patient's finger and his initial SpO_2 on room air is 90 percent. You place a nonrebreather mask at 15 liters on your patient. On auscultation, you hear expiratory wheezing in all lung fields, so you motion to your partner to start the patient on a nebulizer treatment while you initiate IV access. Your partner prepares 2.5 mg of albuterol and 500 mcg of ipratropium bromide in a nebulizer, and tells you that the patient's SpO_2 has risen to 92 percent on the nonrebreather mask. You place a 20 gauge IV with a saline lock in the patient's left hand, and look to see that his SpO_2 has risen to 95 percent after only a couple of minutes of the nebulizer treatment.

By the time you prepare the patient for transport and place him on the stretcher, the patient finishes the treatment. You note a SpO_2 of 99 percent, and auscultation of lung sounds shows that his bronchoconstriction has significantly decreased. You place the patient back on the nonrebreather mask and transfer him to the waiting ambulance. While en route to the ED, you note that the patient's SpO_2 has dropped to 94 percent. You listen to lung sounds, note the return of expiratory wheezing, and prepare another breathing treatment. ■

CHAPTER 11

CPAP—Continuous Positive Airway Pressure

KEY TERMS

Adult respiratory distress syndrome (ARDS)

Apnea

Continuous positive airway pressure (CPAP)

Noninvasive positive-pressure ventilation (NIPPV)

OBJECTIVES

The student will be able to do the following:

▶ List the indications for the use of continuous positive airway pressure on a patient (pp. 70–72).

▶ Describe the importance of proper application and use of continuous positive airway pressure (pp. 70–72).

▶ Describe the technique used to place a patient on continuous positive airway pressure (pp. 73–74).

▶ Demonstrate the ability to place a patient on continuous positive airway pressure (pp. 73–74).

INTRODUCTION

Continuous positive airway pressure (CPAP) is a method of **noninvasive positive-pressure ventilation (NIPPV)** in which positive airway pressure is maintained throughout the respiratory cycle. CPAP can be administered through a face mask, nasal mask, or an endotracheal tube. This chapter will highlight the use of the face mask to deliver CPAP in the field (Figure 11.1).

CPAP is utilized to reduce the work of breathing and increase oxygenation in patients with impending acute hypoxemic respiratory failure. To appreciate how a continuously applied positive pressure would decrease the work of breathing, stick your head out of the window of a moving car and breathe. You will note that the positive pressure in your face created by your head moving through the air makes it considerably easier, almost effortless, to inhale. In the same fashion, CPAP applied through a face mask markedly reduces the work of inhalation, which provides much-needed assistance to those tired patients near respiratory failure.

In addition, it maintains the inflation of atelectatic alveoli and improves pulmonary compliance. The positive intrathoracic pressure that is created can also improve hemodynamics in cases of left ventricular heart failure by reducing preload and afterload. CPAP via face mask is a great tool for those patients who are approaching respiratory failure and may soon require intubation but still have an adequate respiratory drive. In this manner, CPAP can delay and possibly allow you to avoid intubation entirely while initiat-

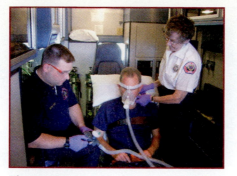

Figure 11.1
Larry Torrey, RN

ing medicinal treatment and awaiting its effects. However CPAP is a temporary measure not a long term one for treating respiratory distress.

CPAP is indicated in patients who are approaching hypoxemic respiratory failure secondary to chronic obstructive pulmonary disease (COPD), asthma, acute heart failure with pulmonary edema, **adult respiratory distress syndrome (ARDS)**, pneumonia, and respiratory insufficiency secondary to trauma. Contraindications to CPAP include maxillofacial trauma, pneumothorax, pneumomediastinum, AMI, hypotension, dysrhythmias, copious secretion production, inability to clear secretions, and active vomiting. Complications with the treatment include accumulation of secretions and gastric distension.

The face mask utilized for CPAP resembles a BVM face mask in that it has a thick rubber seal around the border to promote a tight fit. In addition, two straps secure the mask to the patient's head to further guarantee a good seal on the face, which is required so that the pressure within the CPAP system doesn't escape and lower the effectiveness of treatment. The positive pressure delivered can be "dialed in" by means of a valve that allows for the selection of 0–20 cm of water (cmH_2O) pressure.

The CPAP masks also have a filter to control the FiO_2, or concentration of delivered oxygen. If initiating CPAP in the prehospital environment, a beginning FiO_2 of 95–100 percent is advisable and adjustments will most likely not be necessary prior to your arrival in the emergency department. If transferring a patient with existing CPAP, FiO_2 during transport should match the patient's previously set level. The simplest face masks utilized in the prehospital environment attach to an oxygen cylinder's flowmeter, and can generate the pressures required with 25 lpm airflow. As this system can quickly use up a significant amount of oxygen, it is advisable to have an oxygen cylinder dedicated for CPAP use to ensure an adequate supply at all times.

Application of the CPAP mask is fairly straightforward, but can often feel suffocating to the patient. It is therefore very important to explain the procedure to patients, hold the mask in front of them so they can inspect it, and let them take a few breaths from the mask while you assist them in holding it firmly against their face. After patients get used to the feel of the mask, apply and tighten the head straps while coaching them through the first couple of minutes. The straps must be tightened enough to prevent air leaks while not being so tight as to create patient discomfort. Most patients report an almost immediate sense of relief and ease of breathing after application, so the effort required to make them comfortable with the apparatus is time well spent.

Airway pressure is commonly initiated at 3–5 cmH_2O, and increased as needed to relieve continued dyspnea or to increase SaO_2. Levels up to 10 cmH_2O are common, but levels of greater than 15 cm of H_2O are not and should be approached with caution as the risk of barotrauma increases with higher airway pressures.

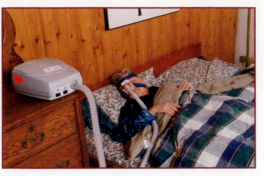

Figure 11.2

In addition to treating respiratory distress, CPAP is often utilized in the home as a treatment for sleep **apnea** (Figure 11.2). Sleep apnea is caused in part by collapse of the upper airway structures during sleep, and CPAP helps to "splint" the upper airway anatomy, preventing collapse and subsequent airway obstruction. In addition to face masks, nasal masks and nasal cushions or prongs are often used.

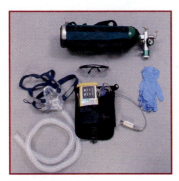

Figure 11.3

▶EQUIPMENT

You will need the following equipment (Figure 11.3):

- ▶ Gloves
- ▶ Goggles
- ▶ CPAP mask and oxygen-connecting tubing
- ▶ Oxygen tank
- ▶ Pulse oximeter

ASSESSMENT

Patients requiring CPAP will present in severe respiratory distress secondary to COPD, asthma, heart failure with pulmonary edema, pneumonia, ARDS, and chest trauma. Signs and symptoms of severe respiratory distress include dyspnea; tachypnea; accessory muscle use; nasal flaring; pale, cold, and diaphoretic skin; peripheral or central cyanosis; retractions; pursed lipped breathing in COPD; a prolonged expiratory phase if air trapping is present; and adventitious lung sounds specific for the etiology. In addition to these findings, obvious patient exhaustion or "tiring out" is a sign of impending respiratory failure and an indication for the application of CPAP.

CPAP requires that the patient is able to produce an adequate respiratory effort and be compliant with the face mask, so those patients in true respiratory failure are not candidates for the treatment. Signs of respiratory failure include bradypnea, altered mental status, decreased level of consciousness, central cyanosis, and apnea. Patients in respiratory failure should be intubated promptly. In addition, assess for the overproduction or inability to clear secretions, as well as vomiting. As the patient's mouth will be covered with the CPAP mask, a risk of aspiration versus benefit of treatment must be performed.

1. Take infection control precautions.

   Rationale: Application of the CPAP face mask will bring your face and hands close to the patient's airway, possibly exposing you to droplet and aerosolized contaminants.

2. Attach the CPAP face-mask oxygen-connecting tubing to the oxygen tank regulator and adjust the oxygen flow to 25 lpm.

   Rationale: 25 lpm of oxygen needs to be supplied to the CPAP circuit to generate adequate airway pressure.

3. Set the airway pressure at 3–5 cmH$_2$O and ensure that FiO$_2$ is 95 to 100 percent (Figure 11.4).

   Rationale: Start airway pressure low and increase it according to the patient's clinical response to avoid high pressures and possible barotrauma.

4. Place the patient on the pulse oximeter (Figure 11.5).

   Rationale: The pulse oximeter will provide objective diagnostic feedback as to the efficacy of treatment.

5. Explain the procedure to the patient and familiarize him with the CPAP face mask (Figure 11.6). Assist the patient with holding the mask to his face for a few breaths in an effort to acclimate to the mask prior to securing the head straps.

   Rationale: Most patients find the face mask at least mildly uncomfortable and suffocating. Explaining the procedure and familiarizing the patient with the mask will help to avoid panic and failure of the treatment (Figure 11.7).

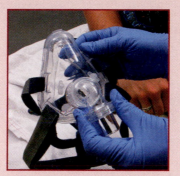

Figure 11.4

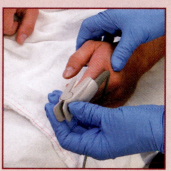

Figure 11.5

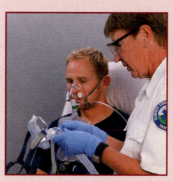

Figure 11.6

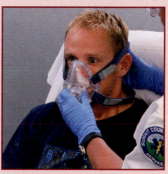

Figure 11.7

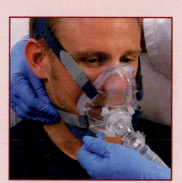

Figure 11.8

PEDIATRIC NOTE:

Newborns and infants, being obligate nose breathers, are often placed on nose masks or nasal cushions (prongs), not face masks.

6. Secure the face mask to the patient with the two head straps (Figure 11.8).

   Rationale: The straps will help achieve and maintain a tight seal on the patient's face.

GERIATRIC NOTE:

If the patient wears dentures, remove them prior to applying the face mask. The pressure exerted on the face with the tightening of the head straps may dislodge them, possibly resulting in a FBAO.

continued...

7. After 3–5 minutes, reassess the patient and increase the pressure in increments of 2 cmH_2O if clinical conditions have not adequately improved (Figure 11.9).

Rationale: Increase pressure in small increments to assure that the lowest pressure necessary to produce improvement is utilized.

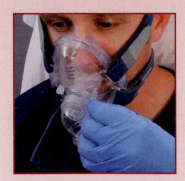

Figure 11.9

ONGOING ASSESSMENT

It is not uncommon to notice improvement almost immediately after initiating CPAP treatment. At 3–5 minutes, perform a primary and focused secondary exam, get a full set of vital signs, and record pulse oximetry. Signs of patient improvement include decreasing tachypnea; decreasing accessory muscle use, anxiety, and work of breathing; and an increasing SaO_2. If signs of improvement do not exist or are not substantial, increase the airway pressure by 2 cmH_2O, and reassess and repeat as needed while not exceeding 15 cmH_2O. If you feel that it is prudent to exceed a pressure of 15 cmH_2O, consult with medical control before doing so.

If your patient shows signs of developing respiratory failure including bradypnea, cyanosis, altered mental status, decreasing level of consciousness, falling SaO_2, or apnea, discontinue CPAP and intubate immediately.

▶ PROBLEM SOLVING

▶ Some patients cannot tolerate having the CPAP face mask strapped to their heads and covering their nose and mouth while they are dyspneic. In such cases, you may have to assist patients by holding the mask firmly against their face without utilizing the straps, as patients find this approach much more tolerable. Use this time to coach and reassure the patient that the treatment is working.

▶ Be alert for episodes of vomiting, as the tight seal and straps will prevent both the vomit from escaping and the patient from quickly removing the mask. Combined with the positive pressure provided, the risk of aspiration in such a situation is high.

▶ Take the time to assure a tight seal, and frequently reassess the seal. Allowing air to escape through a poor seal renders the CPAP unit useless, and demotes it to an expensive simple face mask.

▶ A patient should be sitting upright when receiving CPAP for acute difficulty breathing. If your patient is so weak that he cannot sit upright, you should reconsider your decision to use CPAP and consider endotracheal intubation instead.

►CASE STUDY

You are working as a single paramedic in a flycar servicing a rural community. At 4 AM you receive a dispatch for a reported difficulty breathing. You respond to the scene, and while en route you hear the volunteer BLS ambulance crew call responding over the radio as well. As you pull up to the residence, you see that the EMTs already have the patient on the stretcher receiving oxygen via a nonrebreather mask and are loading her into the back of the ambulance. Even from a distance, you can see that the patient is in respiratory distress.

You get your airway bag, medication bag, and cardiac monitor and walk over to the ambulance and climb in the side door. In addition to the "good morning" from the EMTs, you are greeted with the sound of audible crackles from the patient. You say hello to the crew, and as you bend down and say hello to the patient and ask her if you can listen to her lungs, the crew chief tells you that the patient is an 84-year-old female with a history of CHF, has not taken her diuretics for a week, and experienced an acute onset of difficulty breathing that became worse overnight. You nod in understanding as you auscultate crackles bilaterally to the upper lobes with no air movement in the bases.

Knowing that the hospital is 45 minutes away, you ask the crew to start transport. One of the EMTs looks up from taking the patient's blood pressure and reports vital signs of HR = 118, BP = 142/98, RR = 36 and regular, SaO_2 is 82 percent. You notice one of the local paramedic students on the ambulance crew and ask her to start an IV as you place the patient on the cardiac monitor. You note a sinus tachycardia, and a 12-lead ECG is nondiagnostic for AMI. As the student secures the IV, you note that the patient is using her accessory muscles; is sitting upright to aid her breathing; has cool, pale, diaphoretic skin; and is alert and oriented to what is happening around her.

While you worry about the 45-minute transport to the hospital and think that she might require intubation sometime in the future, you decide that she is a perfect candidate for CPAP now. You ask one of the EMTs to attach the oxygen supply hose to the wall flowmeter set for 25 lpm as you explain the treatment to the patient and set the CPAP pressure for 5 cmH_2O and the FiO_2 for 100 percent, as your protocol requires.

The patient is able to tolerate the mask without much difficulty, and you secure the straps around her head tight enough to ensure a good seal without causing her discomfort. In the couple of minutes it takes to secure the mask, you note that her SaO_2 has risen to 90 percent and her respiratory rate has dropped noticeably. You ask one of the EMTs to take a BP as you place your stethoscope in your ears to reevaluate her lung sounds. After noting a bit more air movement in the bases, you start quizzing the paramedic student about the proper medications and doses you are going to administer to this patient in CHF. ■

CHAPTER 12

Needle Cricothyrotomy

KEY TERMS

Barotrauma

Caudally

Cook® catheter

Cricoid cartilage

Cricoid membrane

Cricothyroid membrane

ENK Oxygen Flow Modulator
Set

Hypoxia

Hypoxemia

Oxygenation

Subcutaneous emphysema

Thyroid cartilage

Transtracheal jet
insufflator (TJI)

Ventilation

OBJECTIVES

The student will be able to do the following:

▶ List the indications for performing needle cricothyrotomy
(pp. 76–78).

▶ Value the importance of properly performing needle cricothyrotomy
(pp. 76–78).

▶ Describe the proper technique for performing needle cricothyrotomy
(pp. 78–81).

▶ Demonstrate the ability to perform needle cricothyrotomy
(pp. 78–81).

INTRODUCTION

Needle cricothyrotomy, also referred to as needle cric, or percutaneous transtracheal ventilation, is used in situations where the need for a definitive airway exists and endotracheal intubation is impossible. This skill is seldom practiced, rarely performed, and often overlooked in situations where it is indicated.

This procedure is indicated when surgical cricothyrotomy is contraindicated, or cannot be performed due to lack of equipment. Needle cricothyrotomy is also indicated when ET intubation cannot be performed due to structural or anatomical causes, or when one is unable to clear an obstruction of the upper airway. Needle cricothyrotomy can also be performed when ET intubation has been attempted unsuccessfully several times and other forms of ventilation, such as BVM or esophageal devices do not allow for effective ventilation.

There are kits available which contain all the necessary equipment to perform needle cricothyrotomy, such as the **ENK Oxygen Flow Modulator Set**. The set contains a **Cook® catheter**, an ENK oxygen flow modulator, a syringe, two lengths of oxygen-connecting tubing, and a transtracheal catheter connection. The Cook® catheter is a 5.0–7.5 cm long, 14-gauge or larger needle with a rigid catheter to assist with correct placement. The ENK oxygen flow modulator is a device that allows manually controlled oxygen flow. In the absence of a commercially prepared needle cricothyrotomy set, a kit containing all of the necessary equipment should be assembled and kept in a readily accessible location, preferably in an airway bag.

Common prehospital methods for delivering oxygen through a needle cricothyrotomy include the use of a **transtracheal jet insufflator (TJI)**, a BVM, or a demand valve. TJI is recognized as the most efficient method of ventilating a patient through a needle cricothyrotomy. The use of a commercial TJI regulator is desirable, as the high-pressure tubing and threaded, metal attachment point can contain the high pressure of a 50-psi oxygen system. If a commercial device is not available, oxygen tubing can be used in concert with a Y-connector to ventilate a patient, but requires the use of a step-down regulator with a Christmas-tree type oxygen tubing connector. In addition, the high pressures in a 50-psi system will tend to blow the oxygen tubing apart from the various connections in the delivery system, requiring the need for constant attention, or holding, by a team member. In addition, a lot of oxygen is wasted in an open system such as this, and depletion of oxygen supply may occur quickly, especially in smaller, portable tanks. As this method of translaryngeal **ventilation** is arguably the most often used in the prehospital environment, it will be illustrated in the following sections.

The use of a BVM to ventilate a patient through a needle cricothyrotomy is common but delivers suboptimal tidal volumes and poor ventilation when compared to TJI. Numerous methods for connecting a BVM with the translaryngeal catheter exist. One such method is to use the adapter from a 3.0-mm pediatric endotracheal tube. Another method utilizes a 3-cc syringe attached to the translaryngeal catheter; the syringe plunger is removed, and the adapter from a 7.0-mm endotracheal tube can then be used to attach the BVM to the open barrel of the syringe. Another method utilizing a syringe connected to the catheter involves placing a 7.0-mm endotracheal tube directly into the syringe barrel and inflating the balloon.

The least efficacious method for ventilating a patient through a needle cricothyrotomy is with a demand valve. A demand valve's flow rate is restricted, preventing the high pressures required to deliver large tidal volumes through the small diameter catheters used in needle cricothyrotomy.

Perhaps the most ineffective method of transtracheal ventilation through a needle cricothyrotomy is the practice of connecting oxygen tubing directly to a wall-mounted oxygen flow meter. This setup simply cannot generate the pressures required to ventilate the lungs, and has been referred to as "apneic **oxygenation,**"hinting at its ineffectiveness at creating true ventilation.

Whichever method of ventilation is utilized, needle cricothyrotomy is not very effective due to the small lumen of the catheter used to allow airflow and gas exchange. However, if a patent airway cannot be obtained by any other means, then needle cricothyrotomy is certainly preferable to prolonged periods of inability to ventilate.

▶EQUIPMENT

You will need the following equipment (Figure 12.1):

▶ Gloves
▶ Goggles
▶ Mask
▶ Stethoscope
▶ Oxygen tank with a 50-psi step-down regulator
▶ Bag-valve mask
▶ Prepared Needle Cricothyrotomy Kit *or*
   ▶ Alcohol preps
   ▶ Povidone-iodine wipes

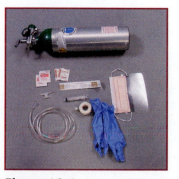

Figure 12.1

- ▶ 14-g or larger IV catheter or cricothyrotomy needle
- ▶ 10-cc syringe
- ▶ (2) lengths of oxygen tubing
- ▶ Three-way stopcock
- ▶ Y-connector
- ▶ Tape or commercial securing device

ASSESSMENT

In theory as well as practice, the assessment of a patient who requires needle cricothyrotomy should never proceed past *airway* when assessing the ABCs. All patients requiring needle cricothyrotomy will exhibit signs of respiratory failure such as bradypnea, decreased tidal volume, or apnea. Cardiac manifestations of developing hypoxia may include cardiac dysrhythmias such as tachycardia, bradycardia, ventricular fibrillation, or asystole, and SaO_2 can be expected to be significantly low. Attempts at BLS airway maintenance and endotracheal intubation should be attempted and declared to be ineffective and impossible, respectively, prior to the consideration of needle cricothyrotomy.

One population of patients who will require needle cricothyrotomy will have a total airway occlusion as a result of foreign body obstruction or edema secondary to an allergic reaction, infection, or inhalation injury preventing the passing of an endotracheal tube. Such patients can be expected to present as unconscious, apneic, and cyanotic or mottled with cold skin.

In addition, the presence of massive maxillofacial or laryngeal injuries may necessitate the placing of a needle cricothyrotomy, as these injuries often deform or obliterate airway landmarks, making identification of the glottic opening impossible. The presence of copious amounts of blood in the airway, which is typical of these injuries, can add to difficulty with intubation.

PROCEDURE: Needle Cricothyrotomy

1. Take infection control precautions.

   Rationale: Both blood and airway secretions will be encountered during the needle cricothyrotomy airway procedure. Gloves and goggles are mandatory when working with the airway, and a mask is a good idea as well.

2. Assemble and lay out all equipment for the procedure. Ensure that the oxygen tubing is connected to an oxygen source capable of delivering 50 psi or greater at the nipple and that oxygen flows freely through the apparatus. If not using a commercial needle cric kit, connect one of the lengths of oxygen tubing to the oxygen source and to one of the upper arms of the Y-connector. Connect the other length of oxygen tubing to the lower, single arm of the Y-connector. Ensure that the three-way stopcock and syringe are easily reachable.

   Rationale: Having all equipment prepared and checked before initiation of the procedure helps ensure the greatest likelihood of success.

3. Identify the anatomical landmarks for needle cricothyrotomy including the **thyroid cartilage**,

cricoid cartilage, and the **cricothyroid membrane** (Figure 12.2).

Rationale: Inability to identify the landmarks due to swelling, bleeding, or anatomical defect is a contraindication for the execution of the needle cricothyrotomy procedure since placing the needle in an area other than the cricothyroid membrane could result in massive bleeding.

> ### PEDIATRIC NOTE:
>
> The necks of infants and children are fleshy and flaccid, making it more difficult to identify the anatomical landmarks. In addition, landmark recognition will be hampered by the small, immature anatomy typical of pediatric patients. You may have to hyperextend the neck briefly, providing no trauma is suspected, to stretch the soft tissue and skin, making the landmarks more pronounced. A smaller catheter is often used in pediatric patients as well.

4. Thoroughly cleanse the skin of the neck overlying the cricothyroid membrane with alcohol preps and providone-iodine wipes (Figure 12.3). This area needs to be as clean as possible before the procedure.

   Rationale: The procedure should be as clean and aseptic as possible since the catheter will be advanced directly into the airway, putting the patient at risk for significant infection if any contaminates from the skin are introduced into the airway.

5. Stabilize the trachea with the thumb and forefinger of your nondominant hand to prevent movement of the trachea during the procedure (Figure 12.4).

   Rationale: Lateral movement of the trachea during the procedure can result in improper placement of the needle.

6. Introduce the needle and catheter into the airway through the cricothyroid membrane at a 90-degree angle. Stop advancement of the catheter when a "pop" is felt, indicating that the needle has penetrated the membrane and is in the tracheal lumen (Figure 12.5). Figure 12.6 is a cutaway view showing the important landmarks of

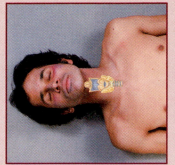
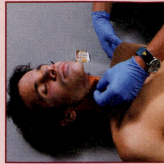

Figure 12.2   **Figure 12.3**

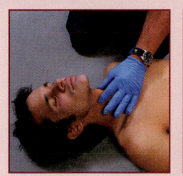
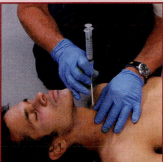

Figure 12.4   **Figure 12.5**

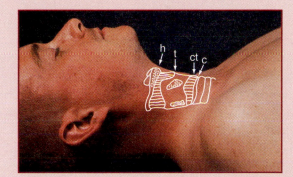

Figure 12.6

the larynx and upper airway: hyoid, thyroid cartilage, cricothyroid membrane, and cricoid cartilage.

Rationale: Very little depth of needle penetration is required to enter the airway (perhaps 1/8th to 1/4 of an inch). Advancement of the needle too far will penetrate the posterior wall of the trachea, resulting in a failed procedure.

7. Attach the syringe to the hub of the catheter, then pull back on the plunger of the syringe to ensure

continued...

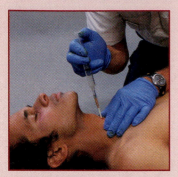

Figure 12.7

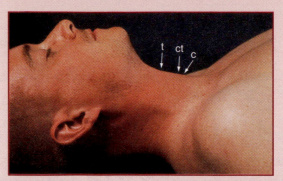

Figure 12.8

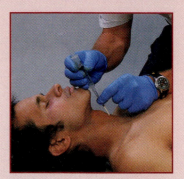

Figure 12.9

that air can easily be aspirated from the trachea (Figure 12.7). If not, remove the needle and abort the procedure. Figure 12.8 is an external view of the anterior neck showing the surface landmarks for the thyroid cartilage (laryngeal) prominence, the cricothyroid membrane, and the cricoid cartilage.

Rationale: The ability to easily aspirate air confirms proper catheter placement into the tracheal lumen.

8. Angle both the needle and catheter 45 degrees **caudally** (toward the feet) (Figure 12.9). The syringe may be left on or removed for this step and step 9, depending on user preference.

   Rationale: The catheter will need to be advanced down into the airway, but doing so after the needle is removed could kink the flexible catheter, resulting in an inability to ventilate. Failure to angle the needle 45 degrees caudally may result in perforation of the posterior wall of the trachea.

9. Slide the catheter off the needle while advancing it caudally until the hub rests against the skin of the neck. Continue holding the catheter with one hand, or ask a partner to do so, until the catheter can be secured in place (Figure 12.10).

   Rationale: This position will help secure the catheter and prevent dislodgement during patient movement.

10. Attach the three-way stopcock to the catheter hub, then attach the distal end of the oxygen-delivery system to the stopcock (Figure 12.11).

    Rationale: This will enable you to ventilate the patient.

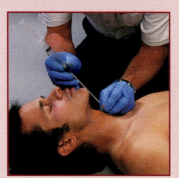

Figure 12.10

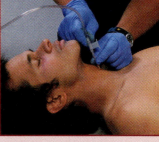

Figure 12.11

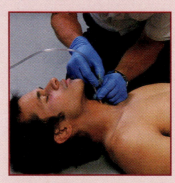

Figure 12.12

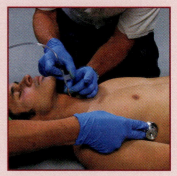

Figure 12.13

11. Ventilate the patient by covering the third arm of the Y-connector or the port on your flow modulator with a finger (Figure 12.12).

    Rationale: Oxygen flow must be directed into the catheter to achieve ventilation.

12. Verify ventilation and oxygenation by observation of chest rise and auscultation of lung sounds (Figure 12.13).

    Rationale: Sufficient volume should be introduced into the airway to observe chest rise.

13. Allow passive exhalation for a longer period of time than was allowed for ventilation. It will be necessary to lift your finger and uncover the Y-connector arm in order to allow exhalation (Figure 12.14).

    Rationale: Both ventilation and exhalation are long processes during needle cricothyrotomy since the diameter of the catheter is so narrow. Local protocols vary, but some systems allow 1 second of ventilation with 2 seconds of exhalation while others use a 1:4 or 4:6 ventilation to exhalation ratio.

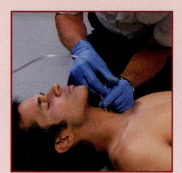
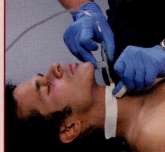

Figure 12.14   **Figure 12.15**

> ### GERIATRIC NOTE:
>
> Geriatric patients are more likely to suffer from emphysema, an air trapping disease that makes oxygen exchange and exhalation more difficult. A prolonged expiratory phase must be allowed in those individuals with any obstructive airway disease resulting in air trapping.

14. Secure the catheter in place with tape or a commercial securing device. In addition, the operator can hold the catheter in place, further decreasing the risk of displacement (Figure 12.15).

    Rationale: Securing the catheter will minimize the chance of having it dislodged during movement of the patient.

15. Observe the insertion site to ensure no edema, bleeding, or **subcutaneous emphysema** develop around the airway.

    Rationale: The presence of bleeding, edema, or subcutaneous emphysema can indicate that the catheter was not properly placed through the **cricoid membrane**, or has become dislodged.

ONGOING ASSESSMENT

Since needle cricothyrotomy is a procedure used only when all other airway attempts have been exhausted, this patient will be critical. Constant monitoring of the airway will be required to ensure that the patient is being ventilated and that exhalation is allowed. Rescuers in a critical situation tend to ventilate more frequently than the patient needs. Doing so in this situation will make it impossible for the patient to exhale completely, resulting in the stacking of breaths and possible **barotrauma** to the lower airways. The anterior, lateral, and posterior neck should be assessed frequently for the presence of bleeding, edema, or subcutaneous emphysema. Due to the high airway pressures generated during translaryngeal ventilation, subcutaneous emphysema may occur even with a properly placed catheter. Subcutaneous emphysema and edema may also develop as a result of a misplaced catheter. Any edema or subcutaneous emphysema noted once the airway is placed necessitates a rapid, thorough reassessment of ventilation to ensure that the airway is patent. The situation should be reported to medical control as the patient may require aggressive airway control immediately upon arrival at the Emergency Department.

In addition to monitoring the airway, continue to monitor the patient's other vital signs. Tachycardia can be an initial sign of **hypoxia**, while bradycardia may develop as a consequence of prolonged **hypoxemia** and hypoxia, indicating the patient is deteriorating.

► PROBLEM SOLVING

► Current literature indicates that needle cricothyrotomy with translaryngeal ventilation can, at best, maintain adequate PaO_2 for only about 20–40 minutes, and hypercapnia immediately develops and rapidly progresses. It is important to recognize that needle cricothyrotomy and translaryngeal ventilation are temporizing measures utilized only until a more definitive airway can be established.

► Proper identification of the anatomical landmarks is imperative since accidentally piercing the thyroid gland, the two lobes of which lay on either side of the trachea at the level of the cricoid cartilage, can result in massive bleeding and further airway obstruction. The isthmus of the thyroid gland connects the two lobes, and is located on the anterior surface of the trachea inferior to the cricoid cartilage.

► Some systems allow introduction of cardiac arrest medications through the needle cricothyrotomy. Check with medical control in your area to determine if your medical control physician finds this beneficial. The efficacy of drugs down the ET tube is poor when the patient can be intubated and ventilated well. It is likely to be much worse when the patient cannot be hyperventilated and when exhalation is so difficult as well.

CASE STUDY

You are working as dual medics in a rural part of town on an ALS transporting ambulance. You are dispatched to a head-on MVC, on a two-lane highway. As you approach the scene, the traffic lanes are completely blocked with deformed vehicles, and the fire department (FD) is on scene. As you get closer you see that the FD has extricated one victim, and is maintaining full c-spine precautions. As you approach the patient, who appears to be in his mid 30s, you begin assessment and realize that his GCS is 3.

You note that the patient has irregular breathing, poor volume, and shows signs of peripheral cyanosis. Your partner inserts an OPA, performs a modified jaw thrust, and attempts to ventilate the patient without success. You reach for your endotracheal tube roll and prepare your equipment for an intubation attempt. You instruct your partner to hold c-spine as you insert a laryngoscope with a Miller 4 blade into the patient's airway. You immediately note that the patient's larynx is crushed and severely deformed and is unable to pass the endotracheal tube. You ask your partner to return to the ambulance, retrieve the 50-psi oxygen system, and open and set up the needle cricothyrotomy kit as you begin to palpate the cricothryroid membrane.

After cleaning the site with alcohol, you stabilize the trachea with one hand as you prepare to insert the catheter. You advance the 14-gauge catheter through the skin covering the cricothyroid membrane, feel a pop, advance the catheter, and attach a syringe to the catheter to aspirate for air. When you aspirate, you get pink frothy sputum in the syringe, but as you ventilate the patient through the catheter with the Y-connector you see adequate chest rise and fall. You auscultate the chest with a stethoscope and hear adequate lung sounds. You ask the team to load the patient onto the stretcher and into the ambulance, where you transport the patient to the trauma center for definitive management of his airway and other injuries. ■

CHAPTER 13
Needle Thoracentesis

OBJECTIVES

The student will be able to do the following:

▶ List the indications for performing needle thoracentesis in a patient (pp. 83–84).

▶ Value the importance of properly performing needle thoracentesis (pp. 83–84).

▶ Describe the proper technique for performing needle thoracentesis (pp. 85–87).

▶ Demonstrate the ability to perform needle thoracentesis (pp. 85–87).

INTRODUCTION

Needle thoracentesis, sometimes referred to as **needle decompression**, is a life-saving intervention for patients with increasing intrathoracic pressure secondary to a developing **tension pneumothorax**. The goal of needle thoracentesis is to relieve the increasing intrathoracic pressure. Needle thoracentesis is not utilized to reexpand the collapsed lung or to evacuate blood from the chest in cases of hemothorax.

A tension pneumothorax can develop from an open **pneumothorax** or a closed pneumothorax. An open pneumothorax most often occurs secondary to traumatic injury and results in the penetration of the chest wall and the **parietal pleura**, which allows air to enter the intrapleural space. A closed pneumothorax can occur in patients with no known lung disease, or can occur secondary to excessive coughing, COPD, or asthma, resulting in the penetration of the **visceral pleura** and the leaking of air into the intrapleural space. Both open and closed pneumothoracies can result in the same outcome; the development and progression of elevated intrathoracic pressure resulting in decreased ventilatory efficiency and decreased venous return to the heart, culminating in decreased cardiac output, respiratory failure, and death unless needle decompression or thoracostomy is performed immediately.

Needle thoracentesis can be performed at one of two different locations on the body. One location is in the 2nd or 3rd **intercostal space (ICS)**, above the inferior rib, in the **midclavicular line**. The other location is in the 4th or 5th intercostal space, in the **midaxillary line**, on top of the inferior rib. For the purpose of illustrating this skill, the 2nd intercostal space will be used. A 14-gauge, over-the-needle IV catheter 2–4 inches in length should be used for the procedure. The catheter is inserted over the top of the inferior rib to avoid the interthoracic nerve, artery, and vein located on the underside of each rib.

After insertion of the needle and successful decompression of the thoracic cavity, many protocols instruct the paramedic to attach a **flutter valve**, a commercial device that is simple and quick to use, onto the catheter left in place. The flutter valve prevents air from flowing into the chest cavity during inspiration, while allowing for the venting off of re-accumulating pressure. It has a multi-sized male coupling apparatus, allowing it to be easily attached to the catheter hub once in place. Another common method of fashioning a flutter valve is to pass the needle and catheter through the tip of a finger cut from a surgical glove prior to insertion into the chest. The collapsible material prevents air from entering the chest during inspiration, while allowing for the release of air during exhalation. Additionally, many systems no longer require a flutter valve at all.

In some instances, the catheter may become clogged with blood after insertion into the chest. This is probably due to a hemothorax within the lungs. A hemothorax usually requires a **chest tube** for relief, and cannot be corrected using a needle thoracostomy in the prehospital setting. If the patient's condition worsens, or respirations become increasingly more difficult, remove the catheter, place an occlusive dressing, and continue to the hospital.

▶EQUIPMENT

You will need the following equipment (Figure 13.1):

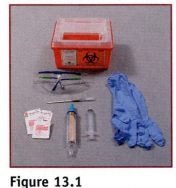

Figure 13.1

- ▶ Gloves
- ▶ Goggles
- ▶ Alcohol preps or povidone-iodine preps
- ▶ 14-g or larger IV catheter, 2–4 inches in length
- ▶ 10-cc syringe
- ▶ Flutter valve or Penrose drain
- ▶ Bulky dressing material such as Kling®, roller gauze, or 4X4 inch gauze pads
- ▶ Tape
- ▶ Sharps container

ASSESSMENT

A tension pneumothorax begins with the development of a pneumothorax, the signs and symptoms of which include tachycardia, tachypnea, shortness of breath, diminished breath sounds on auscultation, and a slightly decreased SaO_2. As more air is drawn into the intrapleural space and intrapleural pressure and volume increase, the lung may further collapse, leading to increasing tachycardia, tachypnea, and difficulty breathing. Breath sounds can be expected to diminish further on the affected side, the patient's skin will become cool and clammy as shock starts to develop, and SaO_2 will continue to fall. As air continues to escape into the intrapleural space, intrathoracic pressure increases, resulting in a shift of the mediastinum to the unaffected side. This will result in a decrease of lung sounds on the unaffected side, as well as a decrease in venous return to the heart due to kinking of the vena cava and aorta within the mediastinum. As venous return decreases, cardiac output decreases, and signs and symptoms of shock will become more severe and include developing hypotension. In addition, JVD will be appreciated as blood backs up the vena cava and jugular veins. As a result, blood is unable to return to the right ventricle. A very late sign of tension pneumothorax is the development of tracheal deviation.

PROCEDURE: Needle Thoracentesis

1. Take infection control precautions.

   Rationale: Gloves and goggles are essential for preventing exposure to infectious diseases when working around blood and needles.

2. Explain the procedure to the patient if the patient is still conscious.

   Rationale: While the procedure will be intimidating and painful, it will also provide significant relief of the patient's respiratory distress.

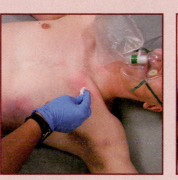 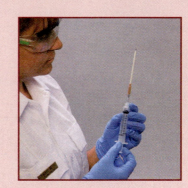

Figure 13.2   Figure 13.3

> **PEDIATRIC NOTE:**
>
> Remember that most significant dysrhythmias in children are caused by respiratory problems. Relief of the tension pneumothorax in a child should dramatically improve his or her cardiac as well as respiratory status.

3. Prepare the site with alcohol preps or povidone-iodine using aseptic technique over the appropriate landmarks of the 2nd or 3rd intercostal space and midclavicular line (Figure 13.2), or the 4th or 5th intercostal space and midaxillary line (Figure 13.3).

   Rationale: Since a needle will be introduced directly into the chest cavity, it is imperative to cleanse the skin as much as possible to prevent intrathoracic contamination.

> **GERIATRIC NOTE:**
>
> Remember that the immune systems of geriatric patients are often compromised. Take special care to cleanse the site and use an aseptic technique throughout the procedure to prevent development of a life-threatening infection.

4. Prepare your equipment. Attach the IV catheter to the 10-cc syringe, and assure that the plunger moves freely (Figure 13.4).

   Rationale: Having all equipment prepared ahead of time assures the greatest likelihood of success.

5. With your nondominate hand, stretch the skin over the 2nd intercostal space at the midclavicular

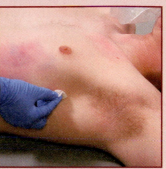

Figure 13.4

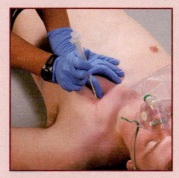 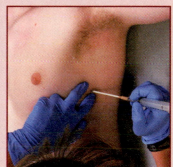

Figure 13.5a   Figure 13.5b

line. Insert the needle at 90 degrees to the chest wall, assuring that it enters the intercostal space over the top of the inferior rib (Figures 13.5a and 13.5b).

Rationale: The needle is advanced over the inferior rib into the appropriate intercostal space because the intercostal nerve and blood vessels rest on the inferior border of each rib. Care must be taken not to injure these structures.

continued...

Chapter 13   *Needle Thoracentesis*   **85**

PEDIATRIC NOTE:

For children, a shorter catheter may be indicated for this procedure. Attempt to measure the depth of the chest wall and choose a length of catheter that is most likely to just barely penetrate the parietal pleura.

6. Verify proper placement of the needle in the **pleural space** by appreciating a "popping" feeling or sensation during insertion, or by easily aspirating free air into the syringe attached to the catheter. In addition, you may witness the syringe plunger move outward as intrathoracic pressure evacuates into the syringe. Pulling the syringe plunger out of the barrel will result in a rush of air as the chest decompresses (Figures 13.6a and 13.6b).

   Rationale: If proper placement is not achieved, the increased intrathoracic pressure will not be relieved.

7. Advance the catheter over the needle until the hub rests on the chest wall (Figures 13.7a and 13.7b). Withdraw the needle by pulling back on the syringe barrel and properly dispose of it (Figure 13.8).

   Rationale: The needle is not left in the chest wall because to do so would increase the risk of lacerating a pleural vessel.

8. Confirm relief of the tension pneumothorax by auscultating the chest for improved lung sounds, observing bilateral chest rise and fall, and noting rapid hemodynamic improvement (Figures 13.9a and 13.9b).

   Rationale: Once the thorax is decompressed, respiratory and circulatory status should improve significantly.

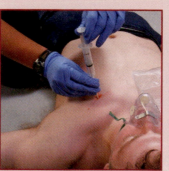

Figure 13.6a   **Figure 13.6b**

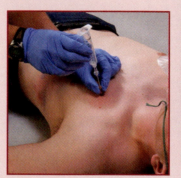

Figure 13.7a   **Figure 13.7b**

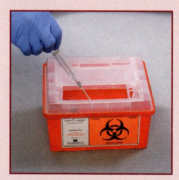

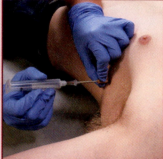

Figure 13.8

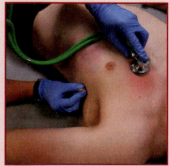

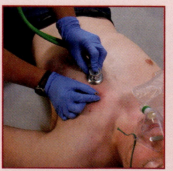

Figure 13.9a   **Figure 13.9b**

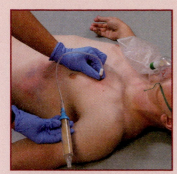

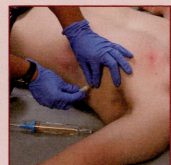

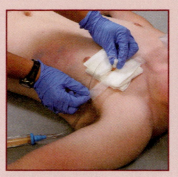

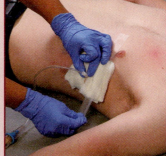

| **Figure 13.10a** | **Figure 13.10b** | **Figure 13.11a** | **Figure 13.11b** |

9. If local protocol dictates, attach a Heimlich flutter valve or **Penrose drain** to the catheter (Figures 13.10a and 13.10b). To fashion a flutter valve, cut the finger off of a surgical glove, then make a small hole at the fingertip. Secure the flutter valve to the catheter hub using tape or a rubber band.

    Rationale: Some systems still require the use of a flutter valve to prevent the negative pressure inside the chest from drawing room air into the chest, possibly worsening the pneumothorax.

10. Stabilize the catheter with tape or bulky dressing as needed (Figures 13.11a and 13.11b).

    Rationale: Catheter should be secured to prevent dislodgement during patient movement.

ONGOING ASSESSMENT

The patient suffering from a tension pneumothorax will be critical, with severely compromised respiratory and possibly circulatory status. Reassessment of all vital signs should be conducted at least every 5 minutes. Assess for continued relief of the pneumothorax by observing an improvement in respiratory rate and effort, equal chest rise and fall, and adequate tidal volume. You should be able to appreciate improved skin color, and an improvement in heart rate and peripheral pulses. It is not uncommon for a catheter to kink or clog up with blood, resulting in the redevelopment of the tension pneumothorax and the need for additional decompression. If the patient remains severely tachycardic, tachypneic, or hypovolemic, look for signs of other injuries, such as further chest or abdominal injuries which might be causing the lack of improvement in condition.

▶PROBLEM SOLVING

▶ Use of the midaxillary or midclavicular landmark location may be dependent upon local protocol. Neither location is preferred, although there are advantages and disadvantages to both. The midclavicular location is a bit high, so a lesser pneumothorax may not be relieved when using this location. However, the location on the anterior chest makes it easier to observe during treatment and transport, and less likely to be dislodged. The midaxillary location is more likely to relieve the tension pneumothorax, which is one reason it is located near where an actual chest tube would be placed. However, the location, which is essentially under the patient's arm, is difficult to observe and likely to be moved or dislodged by the patient's movement.

- Some systems no longer use a flutter valve on the catheter. It is thought that the extremely small diameter of the needle is not likely to allow any significant amount of air to be sucked into the chest cavity anyway.
- If no relief of symptoms is observed after the needle thoracostomy procedure, contact medical control, who will likely order the needle's removal.

▶CASE STUDY

You are working on a paramedic assessment engine coming back from lunch, when you are dispatched to the local soccer field for a patient with shortness of breath. When you arrive on scene you are confronted by several soccer players yelling at you for help. As you get your crew to help control and clear the scene, you notice a thin, tall male about 25 years old lying on the ground rolling around in pain.

When you approach the patient and begin to talk to him, you notice that he can only speak in two-word sentences. You put high-flow, high-concentration oxygen via nonrebreather mask, and grab for your stethoscope. The right lung fields sound clear, but you note that lung sounds on the left are diminished, almost absent. You reconfirm that this is what you hear, and question the bystanders as to what happened. You find out that there was a collision in the middle of the field between two players, and your patient never got up. Further assessment reveals cool, pale, diaphoretic skin, circumoral cyanosis, and a fast, weak radial pulse.

You call for the trauma box, prepare your Cook® Heimlich flutter valve kit, and inform the patient about the procedure you are going to perform. After identifying the proper landmarks, you clean the site thoroughly with an alcohol prep pad, and stretch the skin over the insertion site with your nondominate hand. You insert the needle perpendicular to the chest wall, and feel a pop as you enter the chest cavity. You retract the needle, and hear a rush of air.

Before you even have a chance to listen to the lung sounds again, the patient gives you a thumbs up, confirming that this intervention has helped his breathing. Auscultation of the lung fields reveals only slightly diminished lung sounds on the left side. Your partner places the patient on 100 percent oxygen via a nonrebreather mask as you finish putting together the flutter valve kit, stabilize it with bulky dressings, and place the patient on the gurney. You transport the patient to the ER without any further complications. ■

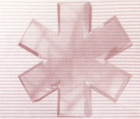

SECTION 2

MEDICATION ADMINISTRATION SKILLS

If advanced airway management is considered life-saving, then IV access might be considered life-sustaining. While the simple task of gaining IV access and administering IV fluid is rarely life-saving, it can buy time for you to get the patient to a hospital by supporting blood pressure and cardiac output in times of fluid loss such as hemorrhage, dehydration, and sepsis.

Frequently, however, medication administration does make a life or death difference. Many of the cardiac medications given to patients experiencing dysrhythmias can either convert the dysrhythmia, or at least prevent the rhythm from worsening into a deadly outcome such as ventricular fibrillation. Preestablished IV access is key to the rapid administration of these emergency medications. While these medications can save a patient's life, they do not come without risk. The miscalculation of a drug dosage can seriously harm or kill a patient. Frequent and regular practice of your IV and medication administration techniques is essential to the safe and rapid administration of emergency medications in the prehospital setting.

CHAPTER 14

Intravenous Cannulation

OBJECTIVES

The student will be able to do the following:

▶ List the indications for intravenous fluid administration (pp. 90–92).
▶ Demonstrate the ability to initiate an intravenous line (pp. 93–96).
▶ Value the importance of proper intravenous line placement (pp. 97–98).

INTRODUCTION

Intravenous (IV) cannulation is a common ALS procedure and involves placing a metal or plastic **catheter** into a vein. The indications for initiation of an intravenous line include the need for blood or fluid volume administration, medication administration, or to obtain a venous blood sample for laboratory studies. In some cases, an intravenous line may be started as a precautionary measure in the event that a patient's condition worsens.

IV lines can be started in both adults and pediatric patients, and include **peripheral** and central venous cannulation. Peripheral intravenous lines are more commonly initiated, and locations for peripheral cannulation include the dorsal surface of the hands, the forearm, the **antecubital** area, the upper arm, the lower legs, and the feet (Figure 14.1). In some EMS systems, providers can establish intravenous lines in the **external jugular vein**, which is considered a peripheral vessel. Central venous cannulation, commonly referred to as a central line, involves the cannulation of deep vessels such as the internal jugular and the subclavian veins and is rarely approved for use in prehospital setting.

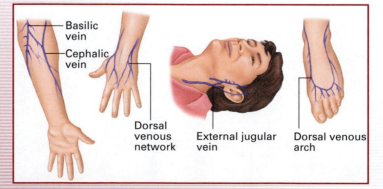

Figure 14.1

Different types of fluids can be delivered through an intravenous line, including normal saline, lactated Ringer's, and D_5W. **Normal saline,** an isotonic electrolyte solution containing **0.9 percent sodium chloride** in water, is the most common prehospital fluid and is used for both medical and trauma patients. **Lactated Ringer's** is another isotonic solution commonly used in trauma patients for fluid replacement, and contains sodium lactate, sodium chloride, potassium chloride, and calcium chloride in water. **D_5W, or 5 percent dextrose in water,** is a hypotonic glucose solution that is often used with medical patients. The small amount of glucose present in the solution can provide calories for cellular metabolism without increasing intravascular volume. Consult local protocol or contact medical control for which fluid is preferred in your area.

Intravenous fluids commonly come packaged in plastic bags of various sizes, the most common in the prehospital environment being 50 cc, 100 cc, 250 cc, 500 cc, and 1000 cc. Medications, such as nitroglycerin, are incompatible with plastic and come packaged in glass containers. Important features on an intravenous fluid bag include an identification label clearly stating the type of solution, the expiration date, an administration set port, and a medication injection port (Figure 14.2).

There are two types of intravenous administration tubing sets commonly used when initiating an intravenous line ."Micro"or "Mini"tubing, which delivers 60 drops per milliliter, is generally used to administer controlled or small amounts of fluid. **"Macro" tubing,** which delivers 10, 12, or 15 drops per milliliter, is used to deliver larger amounts of fluid in shorter periods of time. **"Micro"** or **"Mini" tubing** has a small needle, called a drop former, in the **drip chamber** that limits the flow of intravenous fluid (Figure 14.3). Each **administration set** also has a plastic spike which pierces the administration set port on the IV solution bag that is attached to the drip chamber, a flow regulator that allows you to regulate the flow rates of the fluid delivered, a clamp that completely shuts off fluid flow, a medication injection port, and a needle adapter at the distal end of the tubing that fits into the hub of an intravenous catheter (Figure 14.4).

There are many types of intravenous **cannulas**, or catheters, on the market, with the most commonly used being the over-the-needle type of cannula (Figure 14.5). These cannulas come in different sizes, referred to as the needle "**gauge.**" Different gauge cannulas allow for different amounts of fluid delivery; the smaller the gauge number, the larger the diameter of the cannula. Over-the-needle cannulas are now required to have a safety system that significantly reduces the chances for a provider to be stuck by a needle.

Establishing an intravenous line is not difficult, but it requires diligent practice and some experience to be competent. There may be a time that you are not successful in establishing the intravenous cannulation despite multiple attempts. Don't be ashamed. Instead, consider having your partner attempt intravenous access, reattempt while

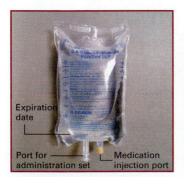

Figure 14.2

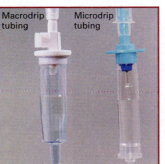

Figure 14.3

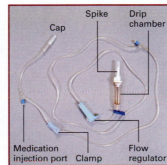

Figure 14.4

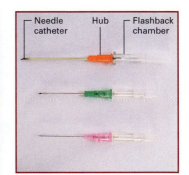

Figure 14.5

en route to your destination, or, if absolutely necessary, consider transportation without an intravenous line. However, do not make so many attempts that you destroy the veins for another health care professional and/or cause the patient excessive pain.

▶ EQUIPMENT

You will need the following equipment (Figure 14.6):

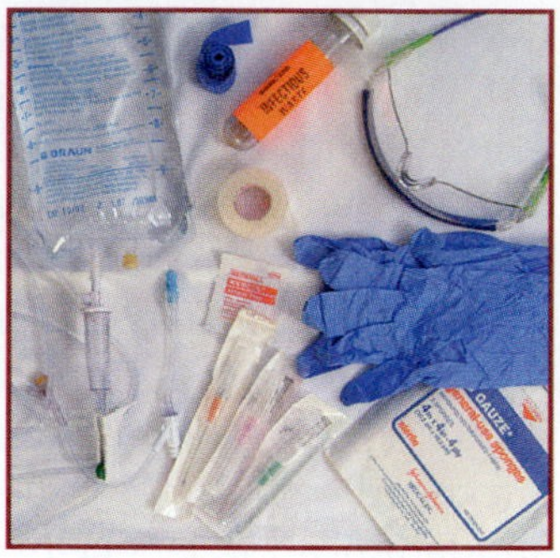

- ▶ Gloves
- ▶ Goggles
- ▶ Tourniquet
- ▶ Alcohol preps and/or povidone-iodine wipes
- ▶ Intravenous catheter
- ▶ Intravenous administration set
- ▶ Intravenous fluid
- ▶ Tape and/or commercial securing device
- ▶ 2 × 2 gauze pads
- ▶ Syringe or blood sample collection device, if needed
- ▶ Hand or arm board, if needed

Figure 14.6

ASSESSMENT

Use appropriate body substance isolation. The patient should be placed in a position of comfort and an initial assessment should be performed, including making sure the patient has a **patent** airway, is breathing, and has a pulse. Level of consciousness and vital signs should be obtained and a focused and detailed assessment should be performed. Any life-threatening signs or symptoms should be treated immediately as they are identified. Intravenous cannulation is usually performed on patients who are dehydrated or in shock and in need of volume replacement, or in those patients who are experiencing a medical emergency requiring medication administration.

The desired site for administration of the IV should be exposed and free of rashes, swelling, edema, bruises, soreness, or any sign of trauma or injury. You should use the **nondominate** extremity if possible so as not to limit the patient's mobility or have the intravenous line accidentally pulled with extremity movement. Pick a vessel that appears straight and free of bumps (valves). Make sure that the vessel will fit the desired cannula. The size of the cannula should be based on the need or potential need of the rate at which fluid needs to be administrated. Do not delay scene departure to initiate an intravenous line. Limit your scene time, and initiate an intravenous line while en route to the medical facility.

Adequate peripheral perfusion is necessary for veins to be engorged with blood and readily accessible. Hypotension, cold extremities, and vascular disease may make intravenous cannulation difficult. Ask patients if they have any vascular disease or diabetes, and do not attempt intravenous access in the feet or hands of these patients unless absolutely necessary, as the poor peripheral perfusion typical of these disease processes increases the risk of infection.

PROCEDURE: Intravenous Cannulation

1. Take infection control precautions.

   Rationale: The needle will puncture both the skin and blood vessel, creating a direct route to blood-borne pathogens. Gloves and goggles are a must during intravenous cannulation.

2. Explain the need for intravenous cannulation, and the steps of the procedure, to the patient (Figure 14.7).

   Rationale: Patients will likely be more cooperative and compliant if they are aware of what is happening and what to expect.

3. Select an intravenous fluid appropriate for the patient's condition.

   Rationale: Different medical and traumatic conditions require varying intravenous fluid. Normal saline is a common fluid for most prehospital conditions, but lactated Ringer's or D_5W may be ordered by your medical control physician.

4. Check selected fluid and packaging for integrity, clarity, and expiration date (Figure 14.8).

   Rationale: All fluid has an expiration date and must not be used if the expiration date has passed. Fluid that is cloudy or has floating particles is an indication of contamination and should not be used.

5. Select an IV catheter appropriate for the patient's condition.

   Rationale: Patients needing large amounts of fluid replacement need large gauge catheters (14 g or 16 g), while medical patients who need only a maintenance or precautionary intravenous line can have smaller gauge catheters (18 g or 20 g).

> ### GERIATRIC NOTE:
> The vessels of many geriatric patients are tiny, which may necessitate a smaller catheter than usual for the patient's condition. A large gauge catheter should not be forced, as it will likely rupture the vein and cause a painful and unsightly **hematoma**. A small gauge catheter is better than no intravenous cannulation when fluid or medications are needed.

6. Select the appropriate administration set for the patient's condition.

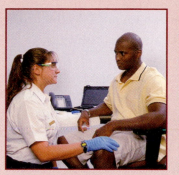

Figure 14.7

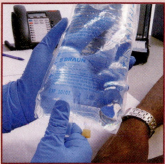

Figure 14.8

Rationale: Macrodrip tubing is required when a large amount of fluid must be infused quickly, while microdrip tubing should be used when a small amount of fluid is to be infused, or when medication administration is the primary reason for the intravenous line placement.

> ### PEDIATRIC NOTE:
> Special administration sets, often called a Buretrol® administration set or burette, may be used for pediatric patients. They contain a special chamber ensuring only the prescribed amount of fluid will be administered to patients, preventing fluid overload in pediatric patients.

7. Prepare the administration set by inserting the spike on the proximal end of the administration tubing into the administration set port on the intravenous fluid bag (Figure 14.9), filling the drip chamber, and flushing the tubing with fluid, ensuring that no air bubbles remain (Figure 14.10).

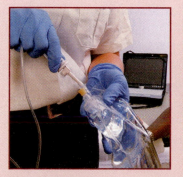

Figure 14.9

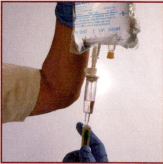

Figure 14.10

continued...

Rationale: Large amounts of fluid in the tubing could put the patient at risk for an air embolism.

8. Tear tape or prepare a commercial securing device.

   Rationale: The intravenous catheter and line must be secured as soon as you determine it to be properly placed in the vein. Any manipulation of the intravenous catheter can cause it to **infiltrate**.

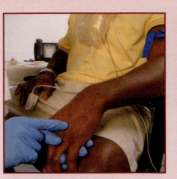
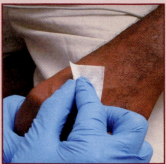

Figure 14.11   **Figure 14.12**

 PEDIATRIC NOTE:

For pediatric patients, as well as those who are combative or have an altered mental status, an armboard should be used to secure the intravenous line and protect it from being pulled out by the patient.

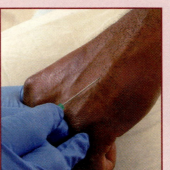
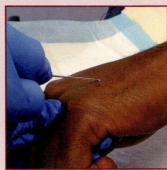

Figure 14.13   **Figure 14.14**

9. Apply a tourniquet proximal to the selected venipuncture site, and place the arm in a dependant position.

   Rationale: A tourniquet will cause the blood to pool in the veins distal to the location of the tourniquet, making those veins more visible and easier to **cannulate**. Placing the arm in a dependant position will further engorge the veins with blood.

10. Palpate the selected vein, and choose the exact site for **venipuncture** (Figure 14.11).

    Rationale: The chosen vein should be as large as possible in the selected area, nonrolling, on a flat surface, and be as free as possible of **bifurcations** (where the vein divides into two branches) and valves. Always begin as distal as possible, in case the first venipuncture is unsuccessful. This will allow you to make a second attempt on a more proximal vessel.

11. Prepare the venipuncture site by cleaning with an **alcohol prep** in widening circles from the inside of the injection area to the outside (Figure 14.12).

    Rationale: Using an alcohol prep in widening circles prevents dragging bacteria on the surface of the skin back over the actual injection site.

12. Stabilize the vein by providing traction to the skin below the venipuncture site (Figure 14.13).

Rationale: Providing traction and stabilizing the vein decreases the likelihood that the vein will roll, increasing the chances of a successful cannulation.

13. Inform the patient that he will feel a sharp, quick pain at the venipuncture site.

    Rationale: Informing the patient of the impending cannulation attempt will decrease the likelihood of her pulling back and disrupting the attempt.

14. Perform venipuncture with chosen intravenous cannula, assuring that the bevel of the needle is upward. Puncture the skin using a 20- to 45-degree angle directly over or from the side of the vein (Figure 14.14). You should feel a "pop" as the vein is entered; ensure that a flashback of blood into the flash chamber is seen.

    Rationale: The flashback is a visual clue that the vein has been punctured as blood is now flowing into the catheter from the vein.

15. Lower the catheter closer to the patient's skin so as to flatten the angle of insertion, slide the catheter and needle 2–3 mm further into the vein, then advance the catheter forward off of the needle into the vein (Figure 14.15).

    Rationale: After entering the vein, the angle of insertion is flattened to prevent the needle from crossing the **lumen** and puncturing the opposite wall of the vein. The needle and catheter are advanced 2–3 mm further to assure that the catheter is fully in the lumen, then the catheter is advanced without the needle to reduce the risk of venous wall perforation.

16. **Occlude** the punctured vein proximal to the catheter with your finger while removing the needle (Figure 14.16).

    Rationale: Once the needle is removed, only the flexible catheter will remain in the patient's vein. The catheter is hollow, allowing fluid to flow through it. However, blood can also flow back out of this hollow catheter when no tubing is connected. Occluding, or putting pressure on, the vein will prevent the backflow of blood onto the patient's arm, clothing, or the floor.

17. Dispose of the needle in an approved **sharps container** (Figure 14.17).

    Rationale: Intravenous needles are sharp and can penetrate a biohazard bag. Needles should be disposed of only in approved, hard plastic containers that can be incinerated.

18. Connect the needle adapter at the distal end of the administration set to the catheter hub (Figure 14.18).

    Rationale: Fluid cannot be administered to the patient until the intravenous tubing is connected.

19. Release the tourniquet (Figure 14.19).

    Rationale: As long as the tourniquet is still connected, no fluid will flow into the vein.

20. Run intravenous fluid for a brief period to ensure the patency of the intravenous line (Figure 14.20).

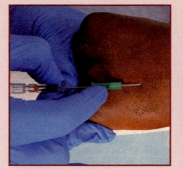

Figure 14.15

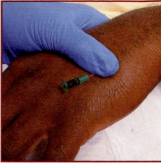

Figure 14.16

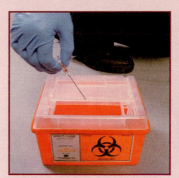

Figure 14.17

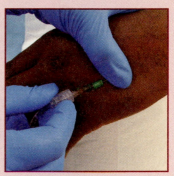

Figure 14.18

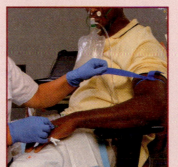

Figure 14.19

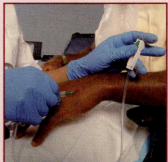

Figure 14.20

Rationale: Sometimes, even when a "pop" is felt and a flash is seen in the chamber, the cannula will not be inserted into the vein properly and the intravenous line will not be patent, or usable. In this case, the fluid should be shut off immediately and intravenous cannulation discontinued.

continued...

21. Secure the catheter with tape or a commercial securing device, looping the administration tubing on the arm and securing it down as well (Figure 14.21).

Rationale: This prevents the catheter from accidentally being pulled out of the vein by patient movement. IV infiltration is a dangerous complication.

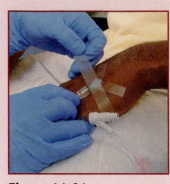

Figure 14.21

22. Adjust the flow rate as appropriate for the patient's condition.

Rationale: Failing to set a specific flow rate can result in fluid overload, a potentially lethal patient complication.

 GERIATRIC NOTE:

Use caution when taping the skin of a geriatric patient, as the skin may be thinner, less elastic, and may easily tear. Skin tears are not only painful, but they open a route for infection that can cause serious complications in the geriatric patient.

ONGOING ASSESSMENT

Intravenous cannulation is, by nature, an invasive skill. While the procedure can be life-saving, it is not without possible complications. Once the vein is cannulated, you must continue to monitor both the fluid and venipuncture site in addition to your patient's condition. Confirm that your flow rate is set properly. If the flow rate is set too low, vital fluid resuscitation may be delayed. If set too high, the patient will receive more fluid than may be safe for his or her condition. Additionally, ensure that the intravenous site remains free of redness, bleeding, leaking, swelling, discoloration, or pain, which can indicate that the intravenous cannula has been displaced from the vein.

If any of the previous signs or symptoms develop, discontinue the intravenous cannulation immediately and do not push any more medications through the intravenous line. A different vein will likely need to be cannulated. Document any abnormal findings on the patient care report.

▶ PROBLEM SOLVING

▶ The most common problem encountered with intravenous cannulation is failure to properly advance the catheter. When entering the vein during the initial venipuncture, a flash of blood should enter the flash chamber. Then, the needle must be advanced a tiny bit further, perhaps 2–3 mm, in order to be in the center of the vessel lumen, before the catheter is advanced. Otherwise, the catheter will often damage the wall of the vessel and come to rest outside the vein, causing an infiltration.

▶ Tape should be torn before the venipuncture is made. One hand will be entirely committed to occluding the vessel proximal to the venipuncture site, making it nearly impossible to tear tape without significant manipulation of the catheter, which nearly always causes **extravasation** of the intravenous fluid.

▶ It is common to forget to release the tourniquet once the intravenous cannulation has been established. Failure to release the tourniquet prevents the intravenous fluid from flowing freely into the vein. Sometimes, providers will actually discontinue a successful IV because they mistakenly thought the fluid was not flowing when actually the tourniquet was still in place.

▶ If it is your agency's policy to draw blood samples for the hospital laboratory from the venipuncture site, you must do so before any fluid is administered to that site. Special blood drawing equipment, as well as simple syringes, can be attached directly to the intravenous catheter for blood draw prior to fluid administration. This practice saves a venipuncture, making the patient's experience with EMS more pleasurable.

▶CASE STUDY

You and your partner respond to an auto/pedestrian accident and find a 34-year-old male lying supine in the street complaining of abdominal pain. Your partner immediately positions herself at the patient's head and holds c-spine stabilization as a firefighter moves to the patient's side to take vital signs and you perform a primary survey. You note that he is conscious, alert, and oriented; protecting his airway; breathing rapidly; and has a strong, rapid pulse. You note that his skin is pale, cool, and diaphoretic, and that he has pain with palpation and a large bruise across the upper quadrants of his abdomen. The firefighter reports that the patient has a heart rate of 132, a blood pressure of 90/60, and a respiratory rate of 28 and regular. You then ask him to administer 100 percent oxygen via a nonrebreather mask at 15 lpm.

While performing a rapid secondary survey you note a fractured right wrist and a fractured left ankle. The abdominal bruising and vital signs cause you and your partner to decide that this is a "load and go" situation, and you tell her to immobilize the patient on a backboard with the fire department personnel while you go to the ambulance to prepare for an ALS workup.

In the back of the ambulance, you prepare the cardiac monitor and your IV equipment. Suspecting that your patient is developing shock, you insert a macrodrip set into a 1000-cc bag of normal saline, fill the drip chamber with fluid, purge all of the air from the tubing, then hang the IV bag from a hook on the ceiling. You tear multiple strips of tape and place them in an area where no one is likely to sit on them, ready two alcohol swabs, and open a 16-g angiocatheter.

The rear doors of the ambulance open, and your partner and the fire department personnel load the patient into the ambulance. You tell your partner to begin transport to the ED, and that you will initiate ALS while en route. You place the patient on the cardiac monitor, and because of the fractured right wrist, you decide to initiate intravenous access in the patient's left hand. You place a tourniquet at the level of the bicep; pick a vein on the patient's forearm that looks big, straight, and without valves or bifurcations; and prepare the site with an alcohol prep. You stabilize the vein by pulling the skin around it taut, inform the patient that he is about to feel a pinch, and advance the needle into the vein.

You feel a reassuring "pop" and note a rush of blood in the flashback chamber. You flatten the angle of approach, advance the needle and catheter 2–3 mm into the lumen of the vein, then advance the catheter off of the needle. You then occlude the vein proximal to the cannula, take off the tourniquet, and pop the protective cap off of the needle adapter before inserting it into the catheter hub. While holding the catheter securely, you reach up and loosen the flow regulator, taking note that fluid runs freely and that there is no swelling or hematoma around the venipuncture site. You then secure the catheter with tape, then make a loop in the administration tubing and tape it to the patient's arm for further security. You then begin to reassess the patient's vital signs, and continue to monitor the venipuncture site for infiltration. You also monitor the patient during transport to the local trauma hospital. ■

CHAPTER 15

Intravenous Bolus Medication Administration

KEY TERMS

Air embolus

Diltiazem

Injection port(s)

Intravenous (IV) bolus

Patent intravenous line

Primary intravenous line

To Keep Open (TKO)

Untoward effects

OBJECTIVES

The student will be able to do the following:

▶ List the indications for the administration of a medication bolus through an IV line (pp. 99–100).

▶ Demonstrate the ability to administer a medication bolus through an IV line (pp. 101–103).

▶ Value the importance of the proper administration of a medication bolus through an IV line (pp. 104–105).

INTRODUCTION

Intravenous (IV) bolus, commonly referred to as IV push, is a method of administering medication through an existing intravenous line. Intravenous administration is often preferred over other means, especially in instances of hemodynamic instability, because of its ability to deliver a high concentration of medication directly into the bloodstream, resulting in rapid distribution and rapid onset of action.

Medications are administered at different rates, depending on the medication that is being administered. Some medications are given rapidly, such as adenosine, while some are administered slowly, such as **diltiazem**.

Some medications used for intravenous administration come packaged in multidose vials or ampules and must be drawn up in an appropriately sized syringe prior to administration. Many intravenous bolus medications come in prepackaged syringes for administration and may or may not have a hypodermic needle on them. Those without a needle are either meant to be used with needleless systems or require a hypodermic needle to be attached prior to use with a traditional system. Many prepackaged syringes come with a needleless adapter that fits over an attached hypodermic needle. With or without a needle, the administration procedure is the same. Prepackaged syringes often require assembling prior to medication administration; the medication-filled tube/plunger is inserted and screwed into the syringe barrel. An internal needle in the syringe barrel pierces the medication-filled tube, allowing for the flow of medication through the external hypodermic needle when the tube is

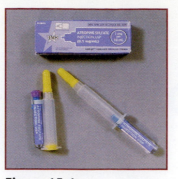

Figure 15.1

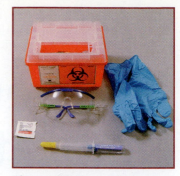

Figure 15.2

pushed into the barrel (Figure 15.1). For the purpose of demonstrating this procedure, a prepackaged syringe will be used.

Intravenous tubing comes with a medication **injection port(s)** on the tubing. The port is usually made of hard clear plastic and has a rubber stopper that the medication is administered through. Some injection ports are needleless with a female adapter. In most cases the port closest to the intravenous site is preferable.

►EQUIPMENT

You will need the following equipment (Figure 15.2):

► Gloves
► Goggles
► **Patent intravenous line** already established
► Prepackaged syringe of medication to be administered
► Alcohol preps
► Sharps container

ASSESSMENT

Use appropriate body substance isolation. The patient should be placed in a position of comfort and an initial assessment performed, including making sure the patient has a patent airway, is breathing adequately, and has a pulse. Level of consciousness and vital signs should be obtained and a focused and detailed assessment should be performed. Any life-threatening signs or symptoms should be treated immediately as they are identified.

Intravenous bolus medication administration is utilized for the vast majority of clinical conditions experienced in the prehospital setting. The assessment of each of these emergencies and situations is much too broad to be included in its entirety in this section, but the advanced provider should be familiar with the clinical signs and symptoms associated with all the disease processes that may require an intravenous bolus administration of medication.

Confirm that the IV site is established, flows freely, and has no infiltration or signs of infection such as redness, swelling, or being warm to the touch. Before any medication is administered, confirm *right person, right drug, right dose, right time, right route* and *right documentation*. Confirm that the patient has no allergies to the medication being administered, and reassess the patient immediately after medication administration for desired and **untoward effects** of the medication.

PROCEDURE: Intravenous Bolus Medication Administration

1. Take infection control precautions.

   Rationale: The preestablished intravenous line rests directly in a vein. Since you will be manipulating that intravenous line in order to administer the medication, you are at risk of an accidental blood-borne pathogen exposure. Gloves and goggles are a must during intravenous bolus medication administration.

   ### GERIATRIC NOTE:

   Remember that geriatric patients often have complicated medical histories, and infectious diseases are common among this population. Because many of the geriatric patients we treat in the prehospital setting may live in an assisted living or skilled nursing facility and in close proximity to one another, they are considered at high risk for the spread of infectious diseases. Do not minimize the importance of infection control precautions when treating the elderly.

2. Explain the procedure to the patient, and confirm that the patient does not have any allergies to the medication being administered.

   Rationale: The patient needs to know that medications may make them feel differently. Helping them to understand the effects and side effects of medications will make those effects seem less frightening when the patient begins to experience them. In addition, you must avoid medications to which the patient is allergic in order to prevent a dangerous allergic reaction.

3. Confirm the correct drug, dose, concentration, and route have been selected for the right patient, and document the information (Figure 15.3).

   Rationale: A mistake with the type of medication, dose of medication, or administration of medication to the wrong patient may at the least undermedicate the patient, and in the worst case prove fatal. In addition, some medications can be administered through multiple routes, such as IM, SQ, and IV. However, only one concentration may be appropriate for a certain condition or route of administration.

   ### PEDIATRIC NOTE:

   Double-check your math when calculating pediatric dosages since very minor errors could result in lethal overdoses in the pediatric patient. Once you complete your calculations, check against a length-based resuscitation tape (see Chapter 25 for more information) or other preprinted pediatric dosing chart.

4. Assemble the prepackaged syringe by screwing the medication-filled tube/plunger into the syringe barrel (Figure 15.4).

   Rationale: Most IV bolus medications will come prefilled with medication and an attached needle that will require assembling prior to use.

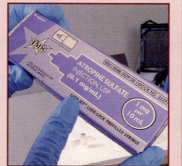

Figure 15.3

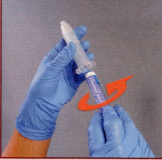

Figure 15.4

continued...

5. Expel any excess air by pointing the needle to the ceiling and gently pushing the plunger to force excess air out of the needle (Figure 15.5).

   Rationale: Excess air in the syringe can cause an **air embolus** in the patient.

6. Cleanse the medication injection port with an alcohol prep (Figure 15.6).

   Rationale: Any bacteria that might exist on the injection port from handling the IV tubing will be introduced directly into the bloodstream of the patient if the port is not cleansed properly.

7. Reconfirm correct medication, concentration, dose, route of administration, and expiration date.

   Rationale: It is possible for medications to be mistaken for each other, misplaced by a helper on scene, or for the paramedic to become distracted in the confusion that is typical of the prehospital environment. This second check immediately before the medication is administered is imperative to prevent lethal medication errors.

8. Stop the flow in the intravenous line by pinching the line or closing the roller clamp above the medication injection port (Figure 15.7).

   Rationale: If the **primary intravenous line** is not occluded above the medication injection port the medication will not flow toward the patient, but will back up into the line toward the intravenous bag.

9. Insert the hypodermic needle into the medication injection port and administer the desired dose of the medication at the proper rate (Figure 15.8).

   Rationale: Most medications have a proper administration rate, either rapid, slow, or at a specific milligram per minute rate. It may be helpful to aspirate for blood prior to administration to ensure IV patency.

10. Flush the intravenous tubing by administering 20 cc of intravenous fluid immediately after the administration of the medication (Figure 15.9).

    Rationale: Some or all of the medication administered will remain in the IV tubing unless fluid is flushed through the tubing, moving the medication forward into the patient's circulatory system.

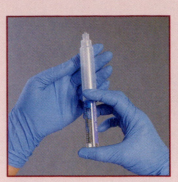

Figure 15.5

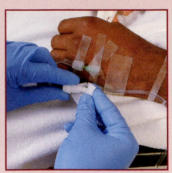

Figure 15.6

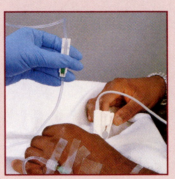

Figure 15.7

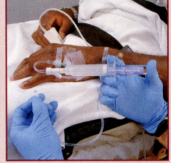

Figure 15.8

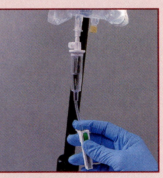

Figure 15.9

> ### PEDIATRIC NOTE:
>
> Even though the pediatric patient is smaller in size, it is still acceptable to use a 10–20-cc flush when administering medications via IV bolus. The purpose of the flush is to remove any medication from the tubing and push it into the patient's circulatory system. Regardless of the size of the patient, the length of the tubing is standard and requires approximately 10–20 cc to flush.

11. Adjust the drip rate of the primary intravenous line back to the desired flow rate or **To Keep Open (TKO)** (Figure 15.10).

    Rationale: When flushing the tubing after medication administration, which is usually done by turning the intravenous line to a wide-open position, fluid overload may occur if the intravenous line is not adjusted back down to TKO or another prescribed flow rate.

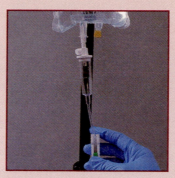
Figure 15.10

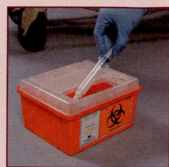
Figure 15.11

> **GERIATRIC NOTE:**
>
> Be especially cautious of fluid overload in the geriatric patient since the incidence of heart failure is higher in this patient population. Heart failure could be exacerbated with a fluid overload resulting in congestive heart failure.

12. Dispose of the prepackaged syringe and needle in a sharps container (Figure 15.11).

    Rationale: The needle will puncture a regular biohazard bag, which could cause a blood-borne pathogen exposure.

13. Reassess the patient for desired effects of the medication and potentially undesirable side effects (Figure 15.12).

    Rationale: A reassessment of the patient is required to note desirable, and undesirable, side effects of the medication. Flushing, itching, paresthesias, dizziness, pain, or shortness of breath are all negative side effects that could indicate an untoward effect of the medication.

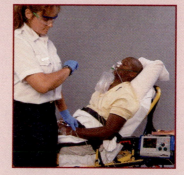
Figure 15.12

14. Document the medication, concentration, dose, time, and effects of the medication on the patient care report.

    Rationale: This information becomes part of the legal medical record and is needed for other providers to continue the patient's care.

ONGOING ASSESSMENT

The administration of medications can alter every physiologic factor of the patient, such as heart rate, blood pressure, and respiratory effort, so it is imperative that vital signs be assessed before and after the administration of any medication. Note any changes on the patient care report, including both positive effects of the medications, such as the dissipation of chest pain following the administration of morphine, as well as negative effects, such as skin flushing after the administration of magnesium sulfate.

Vital signs are an important component of medication administration, and should be measured before and after administration of any medication to determine if the medication had a desirable or undesirable effect on the patient's system. Some medications produce a known drop in blood pressure which might require intervention such as Trendelenburg position or an intravenous fluid bolus.

Additional doses of medication may be required to reach or maintain the medication's desired effect. Continue to monitor the patient to determine if a subsequent dose of medication is warranted. For example, an IV bolus of adenosine may not break a supraventricular tachycardia, thereby requiring a second, larger dose. Alternately, an IV bolus of morphine may control the pain caused by an ankle fracture, but the effects may wear off quickly during a bumpy ambulance transport to the hospital, requiring a second dose to maintain the desired pain management effects.

▶PROBLEM SOLVING

▶ If the rate of recommended medication administration is given in milligrams per minute, the instructions are usually quite easy to follow. However, others are simply listed as "rapid IV push" or "slow IV push." Rapid IV push, in common practice, means as fast as possible. Slow IV push is commonly given over one to several minutes. It is important to follow the rate of administration instructions to avoid a devastating side effect, such as hypotension as a result of pushing the drug too fast.

▶ Some systems use "needleless tubing," tubing whose injection ports do not accept a hypodermic needle. Rather, needleless tubing utilizes standard syringes that twist into place, eliminating the need for a needle on the end of the syringe. The major benefit of needleless systems is the decreased risk of blood-borne pathogen exposure from accidental needle-sticks.

▶ Following the administration of intravenous bolus medication, a flush of 20 cc of IV fluid or normal saline is suggested to move the medication out of the tubing and into the central circulation. An approximation of 20 cc can be administered by opening the roller ball on the tubing and quickly allowing this estimated amount of fluid to flow into the intravenous line. For a more accurate flush of 20 cc, a prefilled syringe with 20 cc of fluid should be prepared prior to the administration of the medication.

▶ It is imperative that the ALS provider check and be familiar with all equipment he or she will be using during medication administration. Fumbling with or misusing a piece of equipment could result in dangerous effects on the patient. For example, if the ALS provider tries to insert a needle into the injection port of needleless tubing, the result will be a hole in, and loss of integrity of, the entire intravenous line. Intravenous access would then be lost, and the patient would have to endure another venipuncture in order to reestablish the intravenous line. Not only is this painful, but it could result in an inability to reestablish the line, and will most certainly result in a delay in the medication's administration.

▶ While not absolutely required, many prehospital systems suggest that patients receiving medication of any kind be connected to a heart monitor prior to and throughout the medication's administration. If a patient is serious enough to require medication therapy in the prehospital setting, he is probably ill enough to benefit from cardiac monitoring as well. The monitor can often provide an early warning of an undesirable side effect in addition to other patient signs and symptoms.

▶CASE STUDY

You respond to the home of a 54-year-old female with a history of diabetes. She is conscious when you arrive but seems to be disoriented. Her vital signs appear to be stable. Her husband confirms that she is a diabetic and that he administered her insulin earlier during the day. He also states that she has not eaten within the last 6 hours. Your partner reports a heart rate of 108, blood pressure of 112/70, respiratory rate of 16, and a SaO$_2$ of 96 percent on room air. You note that the patient has cold, diaphoretic skin.

A fingerstick reveals that her blood glucose is 45 mg/dL. Your partner places the patient on 100 percent oxygen via a nonrebreather mask at 15 lpm and places the patient on the cardiac monitor. You initiate an intravenous line with an 18-g angio-catheter and a macrodrip administration set connected to a 500-cc bag of normal saline. You assure that the line is patent, flows freely, and that there is no evidence of infiltration. You and your partner agree to administer 25 g of glucose via the intravenous line. You clean the medication injection port on the administration set with an alcohol prep while your partner assembles the prepackaged syringe of 50 percent dextrose in water. He hands you the syringe of dextrose as you pinch the intravenous tubing above the medication injection port. You insert the hypodermic needle of the syringe into the injection port and now sure that the line is patent, pull back on the syringe briefly to see blood return into the catheter. You administer the 25 g of dextrose over a couple of minutes, then place the syringe and needle into a sharps container.

After a few minutes the patient is conscious, alert, and oriented. She thanks you for helping her. While your partner is reassessing her vital signs, she states that she has been feeling ill and has lost her appetite and agrees to let you take her to the hospital for an evaluation. ■

CHAPTER 16

Heparin/Saline Lock

KEY TERMS

Aspirate

Cannula

Flush

Hematoma

Heparin

Infiltration

Needleless injection port
  system

Patent

Saline

OBJECTIVES

The student will be able to do the following:

▶ List the indications for the insertion of a saline or heparin lock
  (pp. 106–107).

▶ Value the importance of proper application of a saline or heparin lock
  (pp. 106–107).

▶ Describe the proper technique for insertion of a saline or heparin lock
  (pp. 108–109).

▶ Demonstrate the ability to initiate a saline or heparin lock
  (pp. 108–109).

INTRODUCTION

Intravenous (IV) administration is often a preferred method of medication administration due to the efficacy of concentration, absorption, and rapid onset. Many medications are effectively absorbed only when administered via the intravenous route. In patients with poor peripheral perfusion, the intravenous route may be the only route of administration by which medications can be administered effectively.

Medication can be delivered intravenously without the use of intravenous administration tubing by attaching a small length of tubing with a plug and a rubber injection port to the end of the intravenous **cannula**. Medication can then be administered through the injection port with a needle and syringe. Many lock systems come with a needleless injection port that allows for the attachment of a syringe directly to the port without the use of a hypodermic needle, decreasing the chance of an accidental needle stick. A **needleless injection port system** will be utilized for the purpose of demonstrating this skill.

Two devices provide this direct access to venous circulation:

▶ **Saline lock:** A **saline** lock is used in situations when long-term intravenous access will not be necessary. The device is placed on the intravenous cannula, and normal saline is injected into the tubing to keep the lock open and not occluded with blood.

▶ **Heparin lock:** A **heparin** lock works in the same way as the saline lock but is utilized when the need for longer intravenous maintenance is anticipated. Normal saline will not keep blood from occluding the lock over extended periods of time. Heparinized saline (concentrations ranging from 10 to 1,000 units/mL) is used to prevent occlusion and keep the lock **patent**.

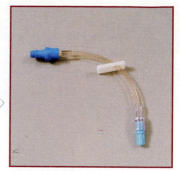

Figure 16.1

Remember that there is no difference in the equipment used between a saline and heparin lock (Figure 16.1), just in the type of fluid used to fill the device. Both the saline and heparin lock can be utilized for medication administration and venous blood draws. When utilized for medication administration, it is important to **flush** the lock with normal saline after administration to ensure that no medication remains in the device. When being utilized for venous blood sampling, it is important to first **aspirate** and discard the saline or heparin present in the lock to prevent contamination of the sample. After use, the lock should be refilled with normal saline or heparinized saline to ensure continued patency.

Saline and heparin locks reduce the costs of establishing venous access. Some studies have shown that the use of a saline lock reduces the risk of loss of the intravenous site due to catching intravenous tubing on an object. Locks also reduce the risk of accidental fluid overload and electrolyte imbalance to a patient with an intravenous line left wide open. Locks are not the best choice for patients who need or have the potential need for fluid resuscitation, as the inner diameter of the lock tubing may be smaller than the lumen of the administration tubing and catheter, and the lock adds to the overall length of the administration system. Both situations serve to limit the flow rate of administered fluids. Because this is part of a closed intravenous system you must always consider the lock port to be sterile, and it should be kept as clean as possible.

▶ EQUIPMENT

You will need the following equipment (Figure 16.2):

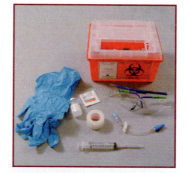

Figure 16.2

- ▶ Gloves
- ▶ Goggles
- ▶ 10-cc syringe
- ▶ 18-gauge hypodermic needle
- ▶ 10-cc normal or heparinized saline
- ▶ Saline lock with or without extension tubing
- ▶ Tape and/or commercial securing device
- ▶ Sharps container

ASSESSMENT

Use appropriate body substance isolation. The patient should be placed in a position of comfort. Perform an initial assessment making sure the patient has a patent airway and circulation. Level of consciousness and vital signs should be obtained. A focused or detailed assessment may need to be performed. Any life-threatening signs or symptoms should be corrected as they are identified.

Confirm that the intravenous site is established and has no **infiltration**. Before any medication is administered, confirm *right person, right drug, right dose, right time, right route,* and *right documentation*. Confirm no allergies to the medication to be administered. Reassess the patient immediately after medication administration for desired and untoward effects of the medication. Constantly check the intravenous site for infiltration.

PROCEDURE: Heparin/Saline Lock

1. Take infection control precautions.

   Rationale: The intravenous catheter will puncture both the skin and blood vessel, creating a direct route to blood-borne pathogens. Gloves and goggles are a must during saline or heparin lock insertion.

2. Explain the procedure to the patient (Figure 16.3).

   Rationale: The patient, especially if conscious, will likely be more cooperative if he is aware of what is happening and what to expect.

3. Check the flush fluid, whether heparin or saline, for package integrity, clarity of fluid, and expiration date (Figure 16.4).

   Rationale: All fluid and medications have an expiration date and must not be used if the expiration date has passed. Fluid that is cloudy or has floating particles is an indication of contamination and should not be used.

4. Draw up 5 to 10 cc of flush fluid (heparinized saline or saline) into a syringe (Figure 16.5).

   Rationale: This flush fluid will be used to fill the lock prior to connection with the patient, preventing possible air emboli. Additionally, the same flush syringe can be used to flush blood out of the lock and to assure that the line is patent with no infiltration once it is connected to the IV cannula.

5. Remove the hypodermic needle from the syringe and dispose of the hypodermic needle in an approved sharps container (Figure 16.6).

   Rationale: Hypodermic needles are sharp and can penetrate a biohazard bag. Needles should be disposed of only in approved, hard plastic containers that can be incinerated. Some systems do allow syringes, with the needle removed, to be disposed of in red-bag trash rather than a sharps container.

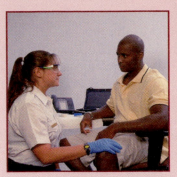
Figure 16.3

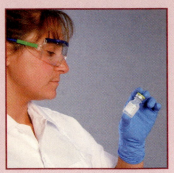
Figure 16.4

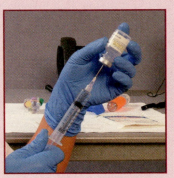
Figure 16.5

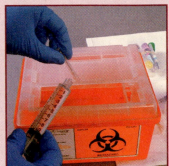
Figure 16.6

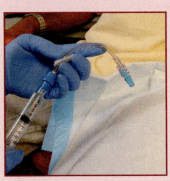
Figure 16.7

> ### PEDIATRIC NOTE:
>
> A benefit of using the lock in a pediatric patient is that the child is less likely to pull the intravenous catheter out of the vein by accidentally becoming tangled in the intravenous tubing. Since locks have, at the most, a couple of inches of tubing, the risk of catching the tubing on a toy or blanket in the crib is less likely.

6. Prepare the lock by connecting the syringe to the injection port and filling the tubing and port with flush fluid (Figure 16.7). Leave the syringe attached to the saline lock.

   Rationale: Any amount of air in the tubing or cap could put the patient at risk for an air embolism.

7. Tear tape or prepare a commercial securing device.

   Rationale: The intravenous catheter and saline lock must be secured as soon as it is determined that the catheter is properly placed in the vein.

Any manipulation of the intravenous catheter can cause it to infiltrate.

8. Select and prepare the venipuncture site and insert the intravenous catheter as you would for intravenous cannulation (see Chapter 14 for the full procedure).

   Rationale: A heparin or saline lock is used in place of administration tubing: therefore, an intravenous catheter must be inserted for access to the vein.

9. Connect a heparin or saline lock to the catheter (Figure 16.8).

   Rationale: The combination of the intravenous catheter and lock provide direct intravenous access for fluid or medication administration.

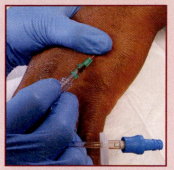
Figure 16.8

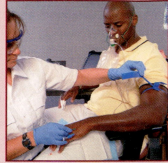
Figure 16.9

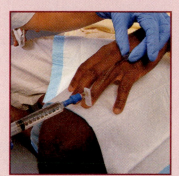
Figure 16.10

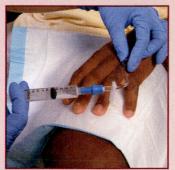
Figure 16.11

> **GERIATRIC NOTE:**
>
> You can draw blood samples for laboratory tests from the lock at this point, preventing another needle-stick to the patient. However, once saline or heparin is infused into the lock, some laboratories may not accept the blood sample, since it may be diluted with fluid. Consult local protocol for lab draws from the lock.

10. Release the tourniquet, which will still be in place from the intravenous cannulation attempt (Figure 16.9).

    Rationale: As long as the tourniquet is still connected, fluid will not flow freely.

11. Aspirate slightly and observe blood return into the lock to confirm that the intravenous line is patent (Figure 16.10). As long as blood is observed in the lock or syringe, slowly flush 3 to 5 cc of fluid into the vein while observing for infiltration into the surrounding tissue (Figure 16.11). Replace the protective cap after removing the syringe.

    Rationale: Sometimes, even when a flash is seen in the chamber of the intravenous catheter, the cannula is not threaded into the vein properly and the intravenous line is not patent or usable. If blood cannot be aspirated or the line does not flush easily, discontinue use and establish a new intravenous line.

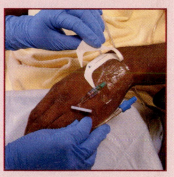
Figure 16.12

> **GERIATRIC NOTE:**
>
> Because the veins of elderly patients are less pliable, flushing fluid quickly can actually cause the vein to fracture or burst, rendering your intravenous line useless. The infiltration will likely cause a **hematoma**. Remove the intravenous catheter, apply pressure to the site, and flush fluid slowly each time you establish a lock in a geriatric patient.

12. Secure the catheter and lock with tape or a commercial securing device (Figure 16.12).

    Rationale: This prevents the catheter from accidentally being pulled out of the vein by patient movement.

ONGOING ASSESSMENT

Reassess the venipuncture site before and after any medication or fluid is pushed through the heparin or saline lock. As with all intravenous lines, a lock can easily be dislodged from the vein during patient movement. Any signs of redness, swelling, hematoma, or reports of pain or tenderness from the patient are indications that the intravenous site has infiltrated, rendering the lock useless.

Since fluid is not always flowing through the lock, blood tends to coagulate around the catheter, which can make medication or fluid administration difficult or impossible. While heparin does a much better job than saline of keeping clots from forming in the intravenous catheter and lock system, a saline flush should always be performed before connecting an intravenous line or attempting to administer medication through the lock. Many systems will have you withdraw and discard the first 3 to 5 cc of blood or fluid from the lock, *then* flush 3 to 5 cc of saline. As long as it flushes easily, the intravenous line is still patent and you can proceed with medication or fluid administration.

▶PROBLEM SOLVING

▶ The first 3 to 5 cc of fluid in a heparin lock should not be flushed into the patient, as this results in the administration of a heparin bolus that may harm the patient. Additionally, that fluid might have clots in it, which would also be potentially harmful to the patient.

▶ If fluid is not flushing easily through the lock, check to be sure a locking mechanism or stopcock is not engaged. Locks with extension tubing often have a clamp of some sort that prevents blood or fluid from backing up into the tubing and clotting there. When the clamp is engaged, it would prevent flow from a syringe or tubing into the lock, appearing as if the lock were occluded.

▶CASE STUDY

You and your partner arrive at the scene of a reported unconscious person and find a 26-year-old female supine on a bedroom floor and responsive to pain only. Her roommate states that she believes the patient had been using heroin earlier in the day. While performing your primary exam, you note that the patient has a gag reflex, is breathing adequately, and has a strong radial pulse. A detailed secondary exam reveals her pupils to be constricted bilaterally.

After placing the patient on 100 percent oxygen via a nonrebreather mask and attaching the cardiac monitor, your partner takes the vital signs and reports a heart rate of 60, a respiratory rate of 12 and regular, a blood pressure of 102/60, and a SaO2 of 96 percent. In addition, a fingerstick reveals a blood glucose of 100 mg/dL.

You and your partner agree that the patient's condition requires the administration of naloxone, but are concerned that she may become combative and pull out the intravenous line once she regains consciousness. To reduce the risk of inadvertent removal of the intravenous catheter, you set up a saline lock while your partner prepares for the venipuncture. You place an 18-g hypodermic needle on a 10-cc syringe and draw up 10 ccs of normal saline. You remove the hypodermic needle, place it in a sharps container, and, after removing the protective cap, attach the syringe to the needleless injection port of the saline lock.

You flush the lock with 5 ccs of saline, and hand the lock and syringe to your partner, who has just performed the venipuncture and removed the tourniquet. He inserts the saline lock into the catheter hub, aspirates blood into the lock, and then flushes the lock with the 5 ccs of saline remaining in the syringe while observing for infiltration in the surrounding fluid. The saline flushes easily without signs of infiltration, so your partner applies a Tegaderm® over the insertion site and secures the saline lock to the patient's arm with tape.

You reassess the patient, determine that naloxone is still indicated, and confirm the medication using the "6 rights" of medication administration. You draw up 2.0 mg of naloxone and administer it through the saline lock, flushing the lock afterwards with 5 ccs of normal saline to ensure that none of the medication remains inside. Minutes later, the patient begins to thrash around and regain consciousness as you begin transport to the hospital. ■

CHAPTER 17

Medication Withdrawal from an Ampule or Vial

KEY TERMS

Ampule

Aseptic

Multi-dose vials

Single-dose vials

Vial

OBJECTIVES

The student will be able to do the following:

▶ List the indications for the withdrawal of medication from an ampule or vial (pp. 112–113).

▶ Describe the importance of utilizing proper technique when withdrawing medication from an ampule or vial (pp. 112–113).

▶ Describe the proper technique for withdrawing medication from an ampule or vial (pp. 114–116).

▶ Demonstrate the ability to properly withdraw medication from an ampule or vial (pp. 114–116).

INTRODUCTION

Medication withdrawal occurs with enough frequency in the prehospital setting that most health care professionals consider it a skill of no great difficulty. However, being complacent or careless during medication withdrawal may result in severe complications or even death to your patient, and as such is a skill that should not be taken lightly.

Before discussing the steps involved in medication withdrawal, it is important to first discuss the difference between an ampule and a vial. An **ampule** (Figure 17.1) is a breakable glass medication container that has a cylindrical base, or body; a thin neck; and a "nipple-like" top. This top piece is snapped off in order to gain access to the medication inside the container. A **vial** (Figure 17.2) is a cylindrical glass or plastic container with a

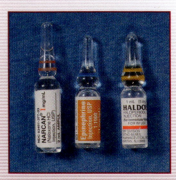

Figure 17.1

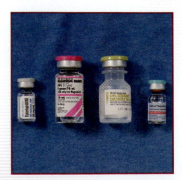

Figure 17.2

self-sealing rubber top. Vials can contain a single or multiple doses of a medication, and are commonly termed **single-** or **multi-dose vials**. The rubber top permits multiple punctures with a hypodermic needle and syringe in multi-dose vials, as well as preventing spilling of the medication from the container.

Once you have determined that you will be administering a medication supplied in an ampule or vial, you will then need to make sure that it is safe for administration. In previous chapters you learned about the "6 rights" of medication administration. Another method for determining safe medication administration is "DICE." "D" stands for correct *drug* or *dose*. Ensure that you have the correct medication that was ordered, and that you know and have the correct dose. "I" stands for *integrity* of the medication packaging. If the integrity of the package is compromised, promptly dispose of the medication in a proper receptacle. "C" stands for *color* and *concentration*. Look at the color of the medication to ensure that it appears as it should. For instance, medications that are normally clear should be so, and not be noticeably cloudy, colored, or have particulate debris. Proper color may be difficult to determine if the medication is packaged in colored glass. In such cases, simply withdraw some medication and inspect the drug in a clear syringe. In addition, inspect the label to ensure that the medication is prepared at the correct concentration that is required for the desired effect. "E" stands for *expiration* date. Make sure that you properly dispose of any medication that has expired. Any time you pick up any medication, you need to DICE the medication or do the "6 rights" to help avoid errors.

Ampules are manufactured in many different sizes and colors. Before opening the ampule, make sure that you gently tap the top of the ampule to remove any solution out of the top of the nipple. It is very easy to cut yourself while breaking the ampule, so be careful. It is best to hold the ampule in one hand using two fingers. With the other hand, use a gauze pad or alcohol prep to grab the nipple. While holding the ampule away from you and your patient, use firm pressure to snap the nipple of the ampule's body at the thin neck, like you would break a twig in half. Make sure that you always break the glass away from you and your patient to avoid injury from glass or splashing medication. Discard the top in a proper receptacle.

The ampule is then inverted, and medication is withdrawn from the ampule with a syringe and hypodermic needle. A vacuum inside the ampule will prevent the medication solution from spilling out. You must make sure *not* to inject air into the ampule, or the medication solution will spill out. Insert the hypodermic needle of the syringe into the ampule with the plunger completely depressed; withdraw the medication from the ampule by pulling back on the syringe plunger. The ampule body should be discarded in a proper receptacle.

Withdrawing medication from a vial requires a slightly different technique after DICEing your medication. It is very important to use **aseptic** technique when using the vial. If the vial still has a cap covering the rubber top, then the rubber top under the cap can be considered a sterile environment. If you take the top off and touch the top of the vial, or the top was previously removed (as can be the case with a multi-dose vial), then it is no longer sterile. In such cases you will need to swab the port using aseptic technique, simply by using a new alcohol prep pad. If you are ever in doubt, swab the port with an alcohol prep. To withdraw medication, the vial is inverted, the hypodermic needle of a syringe is inserted, and a volume of air equal to the volume of solution to be withdrawn is injected into the vial. Injecting air into the vial will aid in the withdrawing of solution, and there is no worry of the solution spilling out, as in the ampule. If using a multi-dose vial, return the vial to its proper location in your medication box or cabinet. If using a single-dose vial, discard the vial in a proper receptacle.

No matter which container you are using, reconfirm the medication order and dose prior to administration, to avoid any complications.

▶EQUIPMENT

You will need the following equipment (Figure 17.3):

- ▶ Gloves
- ▶ Goggles
- ▶ Medication to be administered
- ▶ Hypodermic needle
- ▶ Syringe
- ▶ Alcohol preps
- ▶ Gauze pads
- ▶ Red-bag garbage receptacle
- ▶ Sharps container

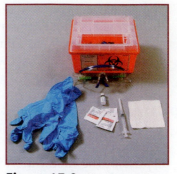

Figure 17.3

ASSESSMENT

It should be obvious that there is no set of assessment findings that are typical for patients requiring the administration of a medication from an ampule or multi-dose vial. Rather, you should have identified the signs and symptoms of a disease or condition that requires the administration of a specific medication that happens to come packaged in an ampule or multi-dose vial. To cover all of these possible disease and condition assessment findings is beyond the scope of this chapter; you should be familiar with all of the disease processes that may require the administration of a medication packaged in an ampule or vial.

PROCEDURE: Medication Withdrawal from an Ampule or Vial

1. Take infection control precautions.

   Rationale: Gloves and goggles are required to prevent exposure to potentially infectious diseases when working with IV lines, medications, and hypodermic needles.

2. Assemble the syringe and hypodermic needle to withdraw medications (Figure 17.4).

   Rationale: Preparing the equipment now will prevent leaving the medication unattended, which could result in spillage or breakage.

3. Ensure that the medication, recipient, dose, integrity, concentration, clarity, and color are correct. Check the integrity of the mediation package and the expiration date (Figure 17.5).

   Rationale: Using DICE to check your medications will help prevent accidents that may contribute to poor patient outcomes.

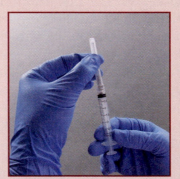

Figure 17.4

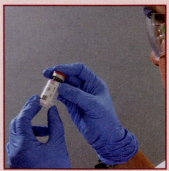

Figure 17.5

PEDIATRIC NOTE:

Pediatric medications often are supplied in different concentrations to prevent accidental overdoses. If an adult concentration must be used, be sure to use proper reference material or consult with medical control to prevent a medication error.

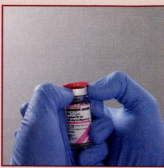

Figure 17.6

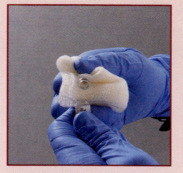

Figure 17.7

4. Open the medication container. If using an ampule, break off the tip of the ampule while protecting your fingers with an alcohol prep or 2x2 gauze pad (Figure 17.6). If using a vial, remove the protective cap (Figure 17.7) or cleanse the rubber stopper with an alcohol prep (Figure 17.8) if the vial has been previously opened.

   Rationale: Care should be taken to exercise aseptic technique when exposing the medication to the environment.

5. Use a syringe and hypodermic needle to withdraw the medication. For an the ampule, invert the ampule, insert the needle into the ampule (Figure 17.9), and withdraw the desired volume of medication into the syringe (Figure 17.10). For a vial, invert the vial, insert the needle, inject a small amount of air into the vial (Figure 17.11), and withdraw the desired volume of medication into the syringe (Figure 17.12).

   Rationale: Air should only be injected into a vial, never an ampule. The lack of a rubber top on the neck of the ampule will cause the medication to spill onto the floor if air is injected into an ampule.

6. Discard the used ampule or vial into an approved receptacle (Figure 17.13).

   Rationale: Glass, especially the broken ampule pieces, should be disposed of promptly to minimize the potential for injury.

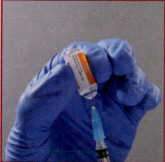

Figure 17.8

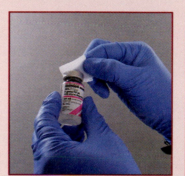

Figure 17.9

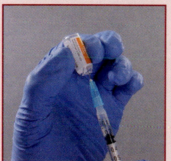

Figure 17.10

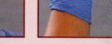

Figure 17.11

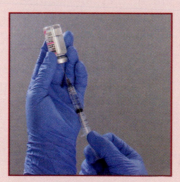

Figure 17.12

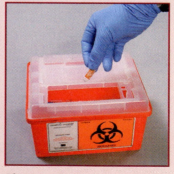

Figure 17.13

continued...

7. Invert the syringe and carefully displace any air accidentally drawn into the syringe (Figure 17.14).

   Rationale: Air injected into the patient's bloodstream can cause an embolus.

8. Reconfirm the medication order and amount withdrawn prior to administering any medication to the patient (Figure 17.15).

   Rationale: Medication orders should be checked at least twice to prevent harmful medication administration mistakes.

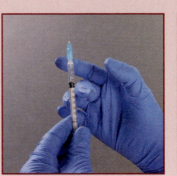
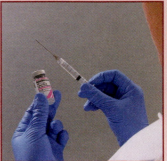

Figure 17.14 **Figure 17.15**

GERIATRIC NOTE:

Geriatric patients are likely to be on multiple medications. Be sure to check which prescription, over-the-counter, and herbal medications the patient is taking to rule out a possible drug interaction with your prehospital medications.

ONGOING ASSESSMENT

Care should be taken to not leave medication unattended once it has been drawn into a syringe. It is a good habit to label all syringes with the name, concentration, and dose of medication. Unfortunately, this is not always practiced in the prehospital setting since medications are usually drawn up and then delivered immediately. However, because you may be distracted with another patient care priority or need to communicate with your partner or the hospital, it is possible to set down the syringe and accidentally confuse it with another.

Occasionally an order for medication will be received, but by the time the medication is drawn up from an ampule or vial, the patient's condition has changed and the medication is no longer needed. Be sure to assess the patient before and after each medication administration. Assess the patient before the medication administration to ensure that the indications for the medication administration still exist, and assess the patient after the administration for desired or untoward effects.

▶PROBLEM SOLVING

▶ While this chapter refers to medications, normal saline is commonly packaged in vials. The procedure is exactly the same, despite the solution not being an actual medication.

▶ The packaging for many medications is nearly identical, despite the concentration. The concentration should always be double-checked before withdrawal from an ampule or vial. Administering the wrong concentration could be fatal to the patient.

► It will be impossible to withdraw some medications from their vials without the injection of air into the vial. Roughly the same volume of air should be injected into the vial as the volume of medication to be withdrawn.

► If you find it difficult to insert the needle into the open neck of an ampule due to ambulance motion or shaking, hold the ampule between the thumb and pointer of your nondominant hand and rest the barrel of the syringe, held in your dominant hand, on the palm of the same hand, steadying it. You can then slowly advance the needle into the ampule.

►CASE STUDY

You are called to the home of a 26-year-old male who is complaining of itching and presenting with hives after eating shellfish. After finishing the initial assessment, and determining that the airway is not compromised, you ask your medical control for an order of diphenhydramine. Medical control tells you to give 25 mg IM, followed by 25 mg IM prn. You go to your drug bag and locate the diphenhydramine, DICE the medication, and note that you have 50 mg in a 2 mL vial. The cap is still on, so you pop the top off as you ask the patient if he has any allergies. The patient denies any allergies, so you withdraw 1 cc of diphenhydramine, cleanse the IM site using aseptic techniques, and administer the medication.

After initiating transport and reassessing the patient, you realize that the 25 mg may not have been enough to relieve the itching and hives. You withdraw the remaining 25 mg, first swabbing the port with an alcohol prep pad, and then administer the remaining medication. ■

CHAPTER 18

Endotracheal Medication Administration

KEY TERMS

Alveoli

Bag-valve mask (BVM)

Capnometer

CO_2 detector

Disposition delivery

Extubate

Intubation

Oxygen saturation

Oxygenation

Ventilations

OBJECTIVES

The student will be able to do the following:

▶ List the indications for medication administration through an endotracheal tube (pp. 118–119).

▶ Discuss the importance of utilizing proper technique when administering medication through an endotracheal tube (pp. 118–119).

▶ List the steps involved in the proper technique of medication administration through an endotracheal tube (pp. 120–122).

▶ Demonstrate the ability to administer medication through an endotracheal tube (pp. 120–122).

INTRODUCTION

In the event that you are not able to establish an intravenous (IV) or intraosseous (IO) access and have an endotracheal (ET) tube properly placed, you can use the pulmonary system to administer a select group of medications.

After administration through the ET tube, positive-pressure ventilation supplied by a **bag-valve mask (BVM)** results in **disposition delivery** of the medication into the **alveoli**, where it is absorbed into the pulmonary circulation across the alveolar-capillary membrane.

Because medications administered by the ETT route are not directly absorbed into circulation, when equal amounts of medication are given IV and ETT, the serum concentration of the ETT route medication is much lower. Studies have shown that the dosage of selected medication needs to be increased from conventional drug dosages to 2 to 2.5 times the recommended dose.

Some medications delivered down an ET tube need to be diluted to increase the volume of the medication. As a general rule, medications administered by the endotracheal route should be diluted with sterile water to a volume of 5 to 10 cc if they do not come prepared as such. This is important because, during administration, some of the medication will adhere to the wall of the ET tube and airways. This will prohibit the medication from reaching the alveoli, and not allow absorption across the alveolar-capillary membrane into the pulmonary circulatory system, reducing both the delivered dose and desired effects.

The absorption of medication through an ET tube is directly related to the quality of **ventilations** being performed. If the ventilations are not adequate or are diminished, the absorption of medications being delivered will be compromised. Note that even with good quality assisted ventilations, patients with severe obstructive pulmonary disease, bronchospasm, pulmonary edema, and other pulmonary pathologies can experience significant decreases in the absorption of medications administered through an ET tube.

The following list notes the most common prehospital care medications that can be administered through the ET tube, and give rise to the pneumonic NAVEL:

- Naloxone
- Atropine
- Vasopressin
- Epinephrine
- Lidocaine

A recently developed device called an endotracheal atomizer has the ability to mist a medication inside the ET tube, allowing for medication to be delivered during ventilations.

Sometimes there is a question regarding the amount of medication that can be placed down an ET tube. Although studies have not confirmed the exact amount of volume that can be placed down an ET tube without deleterious effects, it appears that a significant amount of volume would need to be introduced into the bronchial tree before ventilation is affected.

Recent studies question the quality of this route of administration. These findings suggest that administration down the ET tube should be a last resort to consider for medication administration, utilized only when repeated attempts at peripheral and central venous and intraosseous access have been unsuccessful. Recent studies also show that sterile water is best to use to dilute medications delivered down an ET tube over the use of normal saline.

▶EQUIPMENT

You will need the following equipment:

- Gloves
- Goggles
- Mask
- Medication to be administered
- 10-cc syringe
- 5–10 cc sterile water
- Suction equipment
- BVM
- Pre-established ET tube
- Stethoscope

ASSESSMENT

Initial assessment of the patient who is a candidate for medication administration through the ET tube centers on assessment of the airway. Reconfirm tube placement by observing for proper chest rise and fall, condensation in the tube, an improving

SaO_2 and color in patients with a pulse, and indications of end-tidal CO_2 via a colormetric device or capnography.

Auscultate breath sounds to ensure adequate ventilation and rule out right mainstem **intubation**. Confirm that the patient has good tidal volume with each respiration, as poor tidal volume could affect delivery to and absorption of medication across the alveoli. Check the patient's medical history for pulmonary diseases that could affect medication delivery and absorption.

You must ensure that the patient's clinical condition satisfies the indication requirements for any medication to be administered through the ET tube and that no contraindications to a particular medication exist.

PROCEDURE: Endotracheal Medication Administration

1. Take infection control precautions.

   Rationale: During administration of medication through the ET tube, it is quite possible for secretions to be splashed or sprayed with infectious contents from the airway. Gloves and goggles are a must, and a mask would also be prudent when working around the airway.

2. Confirm the patient's allergies.

   Rationale: The patient will likely be unconscious or sedated if intubated, so allergies may have to be confirmed from a family member, caregiver, or the patient's chart to prevent a harmful medication reaction.

3. Select the correct medication and confirm integrity of the package, proper concentration, clarity, and expiration date (Figure 18.1).

   Rationale: Administration of a medication of improper concentration, or one that is contaminated or expired, can have undesirable consequences for the patient.

4. Determine the proper dose of medication.

   Rationale: Most drugs administered via the ET tube are given at 2 to 2.5 times the IV dose.

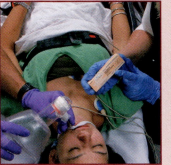
Figure 18.1

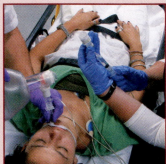
Figure 18.2

5. Prepare the medication dose in a syringe to equal at least 10 cc in volume. Dilute the dose in 5–10cc of sterile water. (Figure 18.2).

   Rationale: Since the tube itself is over 20 mm in length and there is a certain amount of anatomic dead space in the bronchial tree, 10 cc of volume is thought to be needed to ensure that the medication actually reaches the lung tissue.

 PEDIATRIC NOTE:

Since both pediatric ET tubes and pediatric airways are shorter and more narrow, many systems allow less than 10 cc total volume to be administered when giving ET meds to the pediatric patient. 5 cc is a common volume used.

6. Confirm correct ET tube placement by observing for chest rise and fall, noting the presence of end-tidal CO_2, auscultating for bilateral breath

GERIATRIC NOTE:

Though some medications, such as lidocaine, are given in smaller doses to elderly patients, this rule generally does not apply when those same medications are given via the ET tube. Since the absorption of medications via the ET tube is so poor, it is not necessary to half the dose.

sounds, and noting the absence of sounds over the epigastrium (Figure 18.3).

Rationale: No absorption of medication occurs if the tube is misplaced into the esophagus. Only patent ET tubes can be used for medication administration.

7. Suction the ET tube as needed (Figure 18.4).

   Rationale: The medication is less effective if diluted by contaminates in the lungs such as interstitial fluid, blood, or vomit.

8. Ventilate patient with 100 percent O_2 for at least 30 seconds prior to ET tube medication administration.

   Rationale: During the medication administration, **oxygenation** and ventilation will be suspended. Ventilation can saturate the blood with oxygen and prevent a dangerous drop in **oxygen saturation** during the medication administration.

9. Considered pausing chest compressions briefly if they are in progress.

   Rationale: Compressing the chest during medication administration can cause the medication to flow back up the tube before it can be absorbed by the lungs. However, any interruption in CPR can have a negative effect on patient outcome.

10. Remove the BVM and **CO_2 detector** if present (Figure 18.5).

    Rationale: Administration of medication through the CO_2 detector will render it inoperable.

11. Rapidly instill the medication and any required flush directly into the trachea through the end of the ET tube (Figure 18.6).

    Rationale: Move quickly to limit the amount of time that the patient is not being ventilated.

12. Reattach CO_2 monitor and BVM to facilitate the delivery of the medication onto the pulmonary tissue. (Figure 18.7).

    Rationale: The positive-pressure ventilation helps deliver the medication further into the bronchial tree and encourages rapid absorption into the pulmonary circulation.

13. Reconfirm continued correct placement of the ET tube (Figure 18.8).

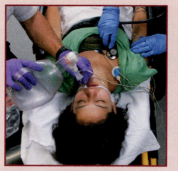

Figure 18.3

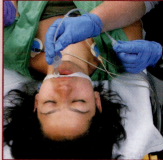

Figure 18.4

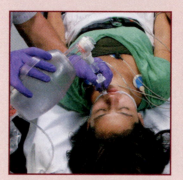

Figure 18.5

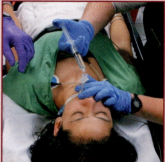

Figure 18.6

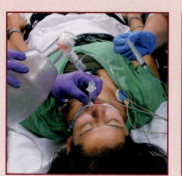

Figure 18.7

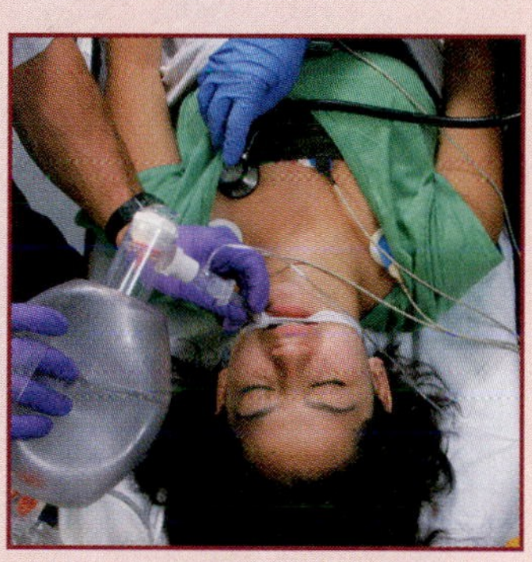

Figure 18.8

Rationale: The manipulation of the ET tube caused by removing and replacing the BVM and CO_2 detector, and by administering the medications through the exposed end of the tube, can cause displacement of the tube from the trachea, which would be a fatal error. Confirm that your handling of the tube did not result in ET tube displacement.

continued...

PEDIATRIC NOTE:

Since the pediatric airway is smaller and more flexible, it is very easy to dislodge the tube. Take special care not to manipulate the tube any more than necessary and confirm continued correct placement of the tube.

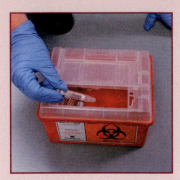

Figure 18.9

14. Resume chest compressions as soon as possible if indicated.

    Rationale: Like ventilations, chest compressions as soon as possible if indicated should only be interrupted during the medication administration and for the least amount of time possible.

15. Dispose of the syringe using an approved technique (Figure 18.9).

    Rationale: If the syringe did not have a needle on the end and is not contaminated with products of the airway, it can be disposed of in regular trash. Contaminated equipment must go in biohazard trash, and needles go into a sharps container.

16. Reassess the patient for desired effects of the medication and potentially undesirable side effects.

    Rationale: Any untoward effects of the medication should be noted and corrected immediately.

17. Document the medication, concentration, dose, time, and effects of the medication on the patient care record.

    Rationale: All medications should be recorded on the PCR to establish a continuum of care.

ONGOING ASSESSMENT

The ongoing assessment of a patient who has had medication administered down the ET tube must begin with airway monitoring. Keep constant vigil on the ET tube, ensuring that the tube remains patent and in the trachea. Signs of accidental tube dislodgement from moving the patient or manipulating the tube during medication administration include lack of chest rise and fall, cyanosis, no condensation in the ET tube, changes on the CO_2 detector or **capnometer**, or falling O_2 saturations. If the tube appears to be dislodged, examine the tube under direct laryngoscopy to ensure that it passes through the glottic opening into the trachea. If you are unable to verify proper ET tube placement with direct laryngoscopy, **extubate** immediately and ventilate using BVM and a BLS airway adjunct until the patient can be re-intubated.

All medications can be potentially life-saving, but also dangerous if administered to the wrong patient or in the wrong dose. Reassess the patient's vital signs every 5 minutes to identify any desired effects of the medication administered as well as to ensure no life-threatening changes to respirations, pulse, or blood pressure have developed as a result of the medications administered.

►PROBLEM SOLVING

► Some ET tubes now come with a medication administration port on the side of the tube. This port allows administration of medication without the interruption of ventilations. It is, of course, a benefit to the patient to have no interruptions in oxygenation or ventilation and to minimize manipulation of the ET tube, capnometer, and BVM.

► It is imperative to deep suction the ET tube prior to administration of any medication down the tube. Medication effectiveness is severely impaired when mixed with airway contaminates.

► Medication administration down the ET tube is not nearly as effective as IV or IO medication administration. Use ET medication administration as a patient management tool, but do not stop trying for venous access. As a general rule, only the first round of resuscitation drugs should be given via the ET tube. IV or IO access should be established as soon as possible.

►CASE STUDY

You arrive on scene and find a 67-year-old male in cardiac arrest. A paramedic assessment engine was on scene first and has been attempting resuscitation for 4 minutes prior to your arrival. The assessment paramedic reports that the patient presented in ventricular fibrillation and was defibrillated without conversion. An ET tube is in place and is confirmed to have good breath sounds and adequate tidal volume. The assessment paramedic has attempted to start an IV with no success. You attempt an external jugular IV and are also unsuccessful in acquiring intravenous access. You then attempt an intraosseous line in the patient's anterior tibial bone and are unable to establish that as well.

You decide that with no IV or IO access and a confirmed ET tube placement, you will administer epinephrine down the ET tube. While you are preparing 2 mg of epinephrine 1:1,000 in 10 cc of sterile water, you instruct the EMT providing BVM ventilations to ventilate the patient with 100 percent O_2 at a rate of 20/min. You disconnect the BVM and CO_2 detector from the ET tube and administer the epinephrine down the ET tube. CPR is performed for 5 cycles of 30 compressions to 2 breaths, then defibrillated and converted into a sinus rhythm with palpable pulses. ■

CHAPTER 19

Administration of Nebulized Medication

KEY TERMS

Handheld nebulizer

Medication chamber

Mouthpiece

Oxygen connect port

T-tube

OBJECTIVES

The student will be able to do the following:

▶ List the indications for the administration of a medication through a handheld nebulizer (pp. 124–125).

▶ Value the importance of properly administering a medication through a handheld nebulizer (pp. 124–125).

▶ Describe the proper technique used to administer medication through a handheld nebulizer (pp. 125–127).

▶ Demonstrate the ability to administer a medication through a handheld nebulizer (pp. 125–127).

INTRODUCTION

A nebulizer is used to aerosolize medications into a mist for delivery directly to the lungs. Medication is then absorbed across the alveolar-capillary membrane into the bloodstream. This is one of the fastest noninvasive ways to deliver medications. Knowledge of the medication being administered is essential. Knowing the indications, contraindications, and adverse reactions and doses are also important.

A **handheld nebulizer** has a **medication chamber** that connects inferiorly to oxygen tubing. Oxygen tubing connects the nebulizer to a medical air compressor or, as in most EMS systems, to a high-flow, high-concentration 100 percent oxygen source capable of delivering a flow rate of at least 5 to 8 lpm. The flow of oxygen through the medication chamber aerosolizes the medication, and the aerosol exits the chamber superiorly into a **T-tube** connector. A **mouthpiece** and flex tubing connect to either side of the T-tube connector. The patient uses the mouthpiece to "breath through" the nebulizer, inhaling the aerosolized medication. Exhalation is evident by the rapid exit of aerosol through the **oxygen connect port**. A nebulizer requires the patient to be alert enough to assist in the delivery process by holding the nebulizer to his mouth and maintaining an adequate respiratory rate and tidal volume.

The indications for use of a nebulizer include bronchoconstriction and the need for humidification of inspired air.

▶EQUIPMENT

You will need the following equipment (Figure 19.1):

- ▶ Gloves
- ▶ Goggles
- ▶ Medication
- ▶ Handheld nebulizer
- ▶ Connection tube
- ▶ Nebulizer chamber
- ▶ T-tube
- ▶ 6-inch flex tube
- ▶ Mouthpiece
- ▶ Oxygen supply tank

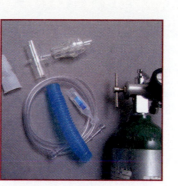

Figure 19.1

ASSESSMENT

Patients who will require medication delivered by a nebulizer will present with respiratory distress secondary to bronchoconstriction. Typical signs and symptoms include dyspnea; shortness of breath; tachycardia; tachypnea; decreased SaO_2; cool, pale, and diaphoretic skin; nasal flaring; retractions; accessory muscle use; and pursed-lipped breathing. Auscultation of lung sounds will reveal wheezing and, in the case of severe bronchoconstriction, severely diminished or absent lung sounds.

After respiratory distress secondary to bronchoconstriction has been confirmed, ensure that the patient is conscious and alert and can comply with simple commands to help with use of the nebulizer. In addition, ensure that the respiratory rate and tidal volume are sufficient to deliver an adequate volume of medication to the distal airways.

PROCEDURE: Administration of Nebulized Medication

1. Take infection control precautions.

   Rationale: Gloves and eye protection are required at a minimum to prevent exposure to infectious diseases.

2. Keep in mind the "6 rights" of patients when administering medications. Ensure that you have the:
   - ▶ Right patient
   - ▶ Right drug
   - ▶ Right amount/dose
   - ▶ Right route of administration
   - ▶ Right time
   - ▶ Right documentation

   Rationale: Following the "6 rights" ensures that proper safety procedures are used for the administration of any medication. "DICE" is another medication verification method used in some systems.

continued...

3. Explain the procedure to the patient (Figure 19.2).

   Rationale: For this procedure to work properly, it requires the patient's assistance. Without the patient's assistance, the procedure is less effective, which may affect the absorption of the medication. The patient is likely to be more cooperative if she understands the procedure. Explain the procedure in a way that the patient can understand what is required of her.

4. Unscrew the lid of the nebulizer chamber.

   Rationale: You are opening the chamber to receive the medication.

5. Add medication as directed (Figure 19.3).

   Rationale: This is where the medication will be housed until it is mixed with the oxygen.

6. Reattach the lid.

   Rationale: The chamber must be closed in order for the medication to be delivered to the patient in the correct dose and concentration.

7. Fasten the T-tube to the nebulizer chamber (Figure 19.4).

   Rationale: This will allow to serve as the conduit between the flex tubing and the mouthpiece.

8. Connect the mouthpiece to one end of the T-tube and the flex tube to the other end.

   Rationale: The mouthpiece will allow the patient to use the nebulizer with convenience and relative comfort.

9. Attach tubing from the nebulizer to the oxygen source. Adjust the oxygen to 6 liters per minute. You should be able to see a mist coming out of both the flex tube and the mouthpiece (Figure 19.5).

   Rationale: The oxygen source is required to aerosolize the medication for inhalation.

10. Ask the patient to sit as upright as possible.

    Rationale: Sitting upright allows maximum expansion of the lungs within the chest cavity.

11. You may hold the nebulizer or ask the patient to hold the nebulizer in her hand and to place the mouthpiece firmly in her mouth. Lips should be sealed tightly around the mouthpiece. Ask the patient to breathe deeply and slowly through her

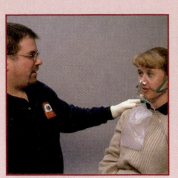

Figure 19.2

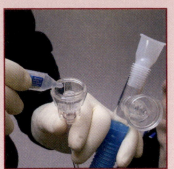

Figure 19.3

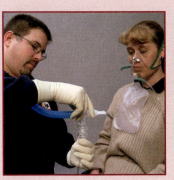

Figure 19.4

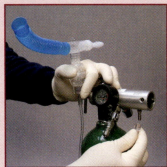

Figure 19.5

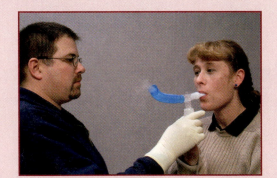

Figure 19.6

mouth (Figure 19.6). At times it may be necessary to shake the chamber slightly to remove medication attached to the chamber's wall.

Rationale: If the patient cannot make a seal around the mouthpiece, medication will escape into the air instead of being inhaled by the patient, resulting in a decreased dose.

12. Continue this treatment until the full amount of the medication is gone.

Rationale: Continue the medication even if the patient is feeling better. The medication chamber has to be emptied before the patient will have received the desired dose.

13. Reassess the patient for desired effects of the medication and potentially undesirable side effects.

Rationale: Any untoward effects of the medication should be noted and corrected immediately.

14. Document the medication, concentration, dose, time, and effects of the medication on the patient care report.

ONGOING ASSESSMENT

Observe the patient immediately after medication administration for desired effects of the medication, as well as adverse or unexpected effects. Additionally, observe for any undesired effects such as itching, dyspnea, or tachycardia. These effects could indicate an allergy or hypersensitivity to the medication. Report these findings to your medical control physician immediately and treat the symptoms present.

Vital signs should be measured before and after administration of any medication. Serial vital signs help to establish a pattern of patient improvement or deterioration as a result of the care you provided en route to the hospital. All patients should have at least two sets of vital signs prior to arrival at the hospital.

▶ PROBLEM SOLVING

▶ If a patient has an adequate respiratory rate and tidal volume for nebulizer use but is unable to hold the device to her mouth, consider removing the oxygen reservoir from a nonrebreather mask and inserting the medication chamber (without the T-tube, mouthpiece, and flex tube) directly into the bottom of the mask. You can then apply the mask as usual, negating the need for the patient to position the nebulizer.

▶ If a patient is in severe respiratory distress secondary to bronchospasm and is unable to produce a sufficient respiratory rate or tidal volume for nebulizer use, consider using the nebulizer with a BVM to deliver the medication. Many BVMs come with a nebulizer port for easy use, and commercial connector devices are available for those BVMs that do not. Familiarize yourself with the equipment your service supplies so you can use it to your patient's best advantage when needed.

▶ CASE STUDY

A 68-year-old female calls EMS after experiencing shortness of breath for 35 minutes. When you and the other responders arrive on scene, you ensure scene safety and don gloves and goggles. Upon entering the house, you find the patient in the kitchen in a tripod position, trying to catch her breath. She has rapid, shallow respirations and is only able to speak in two- to three-word sentences. The patient's husband is on the scene and is able to provide his wife's pertinent medical history.

The husband tells you that she has a 40-year history of smoking one pack a day and was diagnosed with chronic obstructive pulmonary disease 5 years ago. The patient uses home oxygen as needed. Before the current episode of shortness of breath, the patient had just returned from walking her poodle around the block. During the initial assessment, you find a blood pressure of 146/82; heart rate of 126; skin that is cool, ashen, and moist; respirations at 40 per minute with wheezes; and accessory muscle use.

You confirm that the patient is not allergic to albuterol. Online medical control is consulted, and the order is given for 2.5 mg of nebulized albuterol (0.5 cc of 0.5 percent solution diluted in 2.5 cc of normal saline). As you prepare to administer the nebulized medication, you explain the procedure to the patient and confirm the "6 rights" in administering medications (right patient, right drug, right dose, right route, right time, and right documentation).

After adding the medication to the nebulizer chamber and making the appropriate connections, you adjust your portable oxygen source to 6 liters per minute. Upon seeing the mist come out of the mouthpiece and flex tubing, you place the nebulizer in the patient's hands and coach the patient in taking slow, deep breaths while maintaining a tight seal on the mouthpiece. The patient is kept sitting as close to upright as possible while transportation is initiated. Once the medication is finished, you reassess the patient and document the procedure. The emergency department is called with a report and gives an order to provide a second treatment if necessary. The patient remains relaxed and is breathing well, so you elect not to give the second treatment. While transferring care to the emergency staff, you advise them that the patient only received one dose of the albuterol. ■

CHAPTER 20

Intramuscular Medication Administration

KEY TERMS

Adverse effects

Ampules

Aseptic technique

Aspirate

Bevel

Deltoid muscle

Glucagon

Gluteus maximus muscle

Hypodermic needle

Rectus femoris

Vastus lateralis muscle

Vials

Warfarin

OBJECTIVES

The student will be able to do the following:

▶ List the indications for administration of a medication via intramuscular injection (pp. 129–131).

▶ Value the importance of properly administering medication via intramuscular injection (pp. 129–131).

▶ Describe the proper technique for performing administration of a medication via intramuscular injection (pp. 132–134).

▶ Demonstrate the ability to administer a medication via intramuscular injection (pp. 132–134).

INTRODUCTION

An intramuscular (IM) injection places medication into the deep muscle tissue, from which it is absorbed into the bloodstream. The skeletal muscle's rich blood supply assures a fairly rapid absorption rate for administered medication. The absorption of medication is considerably slower than an intravenous injection, but faster than the subcutaneous route.

The most common sites for intramuscular injections are the posterior **deltoid muscle** in the upper arm, the **gluteus maximus muscle** of the buttocks, and the **vastus lateralis** and **rectus femoris muscles** of the lateral thigh (Figure 20.1). A good understanding of the musculoskeletal system is essential for proper injection site location. In most EMS systems the deltoid muscle is the principal muscle used for injection. For purposes of this procedure, the deltoid will be discussed.

The volume of medication that can be delivered via the intramuscular route varies with the muscle group chosen. Up to 2.0 mL of medication can be delivered into the deltoid muscle, up to 5.0 mL into the vastus lateralis and rectus femoris muscles, and 5.0 mL or more into the dorsal gluteal muscle.

Judgment needs to be used to choose the proper syringe depending on the medication being injected. The proper needle length also needs to be considered, and varies depending on the thickness of a patient's subcutaneous and muscle layers. A needle that is too short may result in an accidental subcutaneous administration, and a needle that is too long may strike the underlying bone. Medication administered via the intramuscular

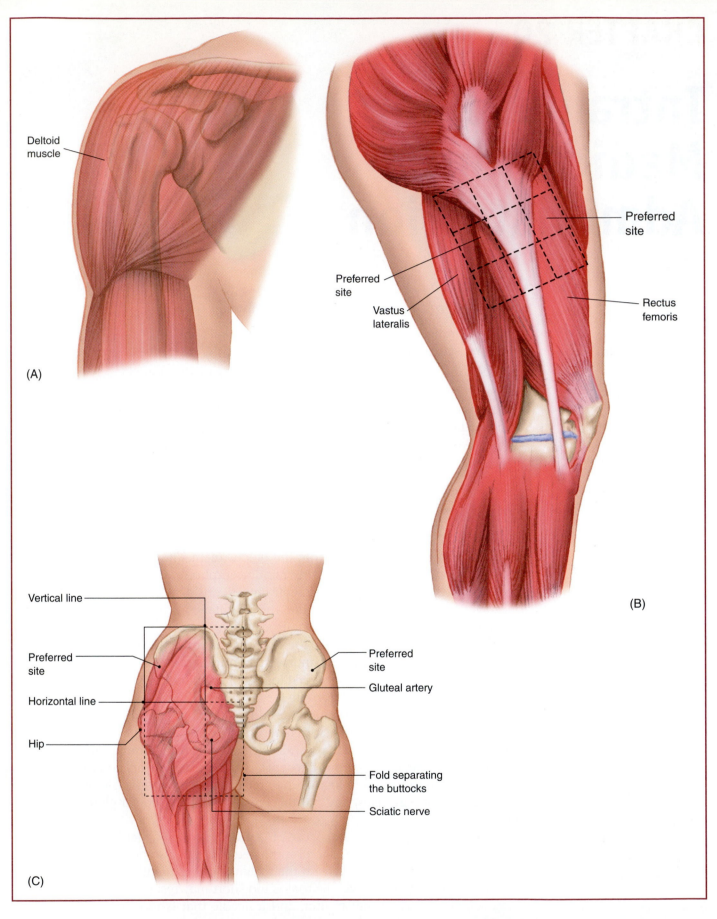

Deltoid
muscle

(A)

Preferred
site

Preferred
site

Vastus
lateralis

Rectus
femoris

(B)

Vertical line

Preferred
site

Horizontal line

Hip

Preferred
site

Gluteal artery

Fold separating
the buttocks

Sciatic nerve

(C)

Figure 20.1

route should be introduced slowly over several seconds to avoid patient discomfort and high intramuscular pressure that could expel the medication through the skin.

Knowledge of the medication being administered is essential. Knowing the indications, contraindications, and adverse reactions and doses is important to assure proper patient care and avoid possible undesirable outcomes.

▶EQUIPMENT

You will need the following equipment (Figure 20.2):

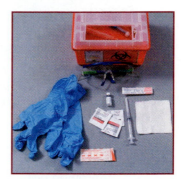
Figure 20.2

- ▶ Gloves
- ▶ Goggles
- ▶ Medication to be administered
- ▶ 3-cc syringe
- ▶ 18-gauge hypodermic needle to withdraw medication
- ▶ 20- to 22-gauge, 3/8"-1" hypodermic needle for medication administration
- ▶ Alcohol preps
- ▶ 2×2 gauze pads
- ▶ Bandage
- ▶ Sharps container

ASSESSMENT

Use appropriate body substance isolation. The patient should be placed in a position of comfort and an initial assessment should be performed, including making sure the patient has a patent airway, is breathing, and has a pulse. Level of consciousness and vital signs should be obtained and a focused and detailed assessment should be performed. Any life-threatening signs or symptoms should be treated immediately as they are identified.

Intramuscular medication administration is utilized for a limited number of clinical conditions in the prehospital setting, and may include but not be limited to the administration of **glucagon** in cases of hypoglycemia, midazolam for seizures or sedation, and morphine for analgesia. The assessment of each of these emergencies and situations is much too broad to be included in their entirety in this section, but the paramedic should be familiar with the clinical signs and symptoms associated with all the disease processes that may require an intramuscular administration of medication.

The desired site for administration should be exposed and free of superficial blood vessels, rashes, swelling, edema, bruises, and soreness. Adequate peripheral perfusion must be assured prior to intramuscular administration or the delivered medication may not be sufficiently absorbed into general circulation. If adequate perfusion is not present, an alternative administration route should be considered, such as intravenous administration.

Before any medication is administered, confirm *right person, right drug, right dose, right time, right route,* and *right documentation.* Confirm that the patient has no allergies to the medication being administered, and reassess the patient immediately after medication administration for desired and untoward effects.

PROCEDURE: Intramuscular Medication Administration

1. Take infection control precautions.

   Rationale: It is possible to accidentally enter a vein when administering medication intramuscularly, resulting in a splash or spill of blood. Gloves and goggles should be worn during the intramuscular injection to avoid a blood-borne pathogen exposure.

2. Explain the procedure to the patient, and confirm that the patient does not have an allergy to the medication being administered.

   Rationale: The intramuscular injection is going to hurt, with the feeling being similar to a bee sting. Proper planning will minimize the chances of the patient moving or pulling away, causing the injection to have to be repeated. A known allergy to a drug is a contraindication to any medication administration.

   > ### PEDIATRIC NOTE:
   >
   > The pediatric patient may not be able to tell you his or her allergies. While it is always a good idea to ask the child first, confirm the information with a parent or caregiver since an allergic reaction could be life threatening.

3. Confirm the right drug, dose, concentration, and route have been selected for the right patient, and document the information (Figure 20.3).

   Rationale: A mistake with the type of medication, dose of medication, or administration of medication to the wrong patient may at the least undermedicate the patient, and in the worst case prove fatal. In addition, some medications can be administered through multiple routes, such as IM, SQ, and IV. However, only one concentration may be appropriate for a certain condition or route of administration.

4. Assemble the 18-g needle and 3-cc syringe (Figure 20.4).

   Rationale: Most intramuscular medications will not come prefilled with medication and an attached needle, but are often supplied in **ampules** or **vials** and must be drawn into a syringe using a **hypodermic needle**.

5. Withdraw the proper amount of medication from the ampule or vial into the syringe (see Chapter 17 for the entire procedure) (Figure 20.5).

   Rationale: When the medication does not come as a prefilled syringe, it must be drawn into the syringe with a hypodermic needle. Drawing up only the proper amount to be administered can help prevent accidental overdoses since only the desired dose will be in the syringe.

6. Change the hypodermic needle from the one used to draw up the medication to the proper size for intramuscular injection.

   Rationale: Often, a larger needle (18 g) is used to draw medication into the syringe than is necessary for injection (20–22 g). Additionally, changing needles helps to ensure **aseptic technique**.

7. Expel any excess air by pointing the needle to the ceiling and gently pushing excess air out of the needle. Be careful not to push an excessive amount of medication out the end of the needle, or your carefully calculated dose will be incorrect (Figure 20.6).

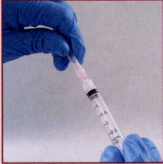

Figure 20.3

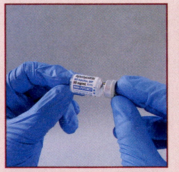

Figure 20.4

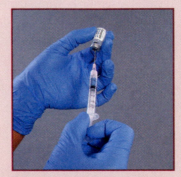

Figure 20.5

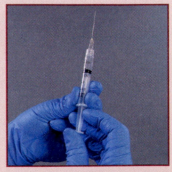

Figure 20.6

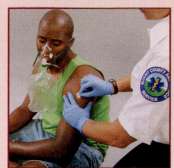

Figure 20.7

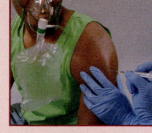

Figure 20.8

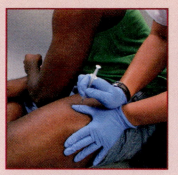

Figure 20.9

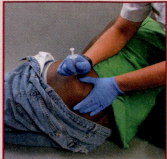

Figure 20.10

Rationale: Excess air in the syringe can cause an air embolus in the patient.

8. Reconfirm correct medication, concentration, dose, route of administration, and expiration date.

   Rationale: It is possible for medications to be mistaken for another, misplaced by a helper on scene, or for the paramedic to become distracted in the confusion that is typical of the prehospital environment. This second check immediately before the medication is administered is imperative to prevent lethal medication errors.

9. Select the appropriate injection site using proper landmarks; in this case, the deltoid muscle will be utilized.

   Rationale: Careful consideration should be given to choosing the injection site. Since the intramuscular injection is deep, a site with adequate muscle tissue must be selected to prevent hitting the bone or other underlying structures.

PEDIATRIC NOTE:

While the deltoid is a common intramuscular injection site for adults, the muscle there is often underdeveloped in the pediatric patient. The quadriceps muscle or gluteus is a better choice for intramuscular injections in a child or infant.

10. Prepare the injection site by cleaning with an alcohol prep in widening circles from the inside of the injection area to the outside (Figure 20.7).

    Rationale: Using an alcohol prep in widening circles prevents dragging bacteria on the surface of the skin back over the actual injection site.

GERIATRIC NOTE:

The geriatric patient is more likely to be immobile or need assistance with activities of daily living, which often means that grooming and bathing become less frequent. This often means more contaminates on the surface of the skin, including dead skin cells, which need to be thoroughly removed. Don't be afraid to use multiple alcohol preps to clean the injection site if needed.

11. Spread the skin taut around the injection site without contaminating the site.

    Rationale: Pulling skin taut will help the needle penetrate smoothly into the underlying muscle.

12. Insert the needle quickly at a 90° angle, with the **bevel** up (Figures 20.8, 20.9, and 20.10).

    Rationale: The angle of injection helps deliver the medication to the underlying muscle, rather than the subcutaneous tissue (Figure 20.11). Figure 20.12 diagrams intramuscular injection.

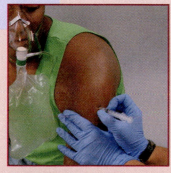

Figure 20.11

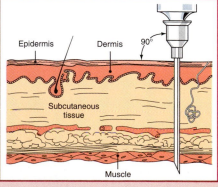

Figure 20.12

continued...

13. **Aspirate** the syringe, confirming that no blood is present in the syringe (Figure 20.13).

    Rationale: Blood in the syringe would indicate that the needle has accidentally been placed in a vein, rather than the muscle. If this occurs, discontinue the procedure and begin again in another location.

14. Inject the medication slowly, over several seconds (Figure 20.14).

    Rationale: Patients can often feel the medication entering the muscle. Administering the medication too quickly can cause unnecessary discomfort.

15. Apply counter-pressure with an alcohol prep or gauze pad and quickly withdraw the needle.

    Rationale: Counter-pressure minimizes discomfort caused by movement of the needle.

16. Apply direct pressure over the injection site with a gauze pad to control any bleeding. Apply a bandage if necessary (Figure 20.15).

    Rationale: Very minimal bleeding should occur, but is possible; like any bleeding, it should be controlled.

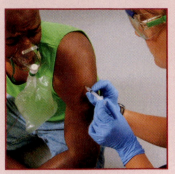

Figure 20.13

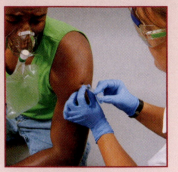

Figure 20.14

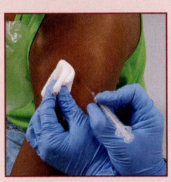

Figure 20.15

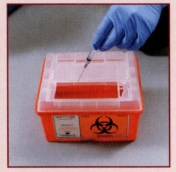

Figure 20.16

 GERIATRIC NOTE:

> Many geriatric patients will be taking an aspirin a day for good heart health or actually be on a blood thinning medication such as **warfarin**, which keeps their blood from clotting. You may observe more serious bleeding even from a minor puncture such as the intramuscular injection. Be sure to hold direct pressure until the bleeding stops, which could be as long as 5–7 minutes.

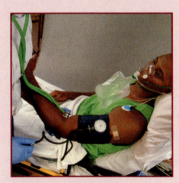

Figure 20.17

17. Dispose of equipment in an approved sharps container (Figure 20.16).

    Rationale: The syringe will definitely have a needle attached and must be placed in a sharps container to prevent an accidental needle-stick.

18. Reassess the patient for desired effects of the medication and potentially undesirable side effects (Figure 20.17).

    Rationale: Any untoward effects of the medication should be noted and corrected immediately.

19. Document the medication, concentration, dose, time, and effects of the medication on the patient care report.

Observe the patient immediately after medication administration for desired effects of the medication, as well as adverse or unexpected effects. Manage the symptoms of any **adverse effects**. For example, administration of glucagon should improve the level of consciousness of a diabetic patient suffering from hypoglycemia; however, this same effect may also cause the patient to be combative before he is fully oriented. The improvement in level of consciousness is desired, but the undesirable, yet expected side effect of agitation must also be anticipated. Additionally, observe for any undesired effects such as itching, dyspnea, or tachycardia. These effects could indicate an allergy or hypersensitivity to the medication. Report these findings to your medical control physician immediately and treat the symptoms present.

Vital signs should be measured before and after administration of any medication. Serial vital signs help to establish a pattern of patient improvement or deterioration as a result of the care you provided en route to the hospital. All patients should have at least two sets of vital signs prior to their arrival at the hospital.

▶ PROBLEM SOLVING

▶ Intramuscular injection is not the best choice for poorly perfusing patients. Since blood is shunted from the skin and skeletal muscles during a shock state, medications administered via the intramuscular route may have delayed absorption times.

▶ While the deltoid muscle is a common site for prehospital intramuscular injections, other deep muscle tissue is appropriate as well such as the gluteus maximus, rectus femoris, and vastus lateralis muscles. The deltoid is commonly chosen because it involves the least amount of disrobing for the patient and provides easier access for the provider. However, in patients with upper extremity abnormalities such as amputations, other approved intramuscular sites work just as well.

▶ Be sure to choose the proper needle length and gauge for the site chosen. Most intramuscular medications need to be given deep into the muscle. A 1″ needle might suffice for the deltoid, but a 1.5″ or 2″ needle might be required for a gluteal injection if much adipose tissue rests over the muscle.

▶ While not absolutely required, many prehospital systems suggest that patients receiving medication of any kind be connected to a heart monitor prior to and throughout the administration of the medication. If a patient is serious enough to require medication therapy in the prehospital setting, he is probably ill enough to benefit from cardiac monitoring as well. The monitor can often provide an early warning of an undesirable side effect in addition to other patient signs and symptoms.

▶ CASE STUDY

It's 8 am, and you and your partner are called to the home of a 54-year-old female who was found unconscious in bed by her daughter. As the patient's daughter leads you back to the patient's bedroom, she informs you that her mother is an insulin-dependant diabetic and has been sick for the past few days. She went to bed early last night after having a light dinner and was found unconscious a few minutes ago.

You arrive at the patient's bedside and note that she is lying supine in bed with snoring respirations. Your partner immediately performs a head tilt-chin lift, which relieves the snoring. As you place the patient on 100 percent oxygen via a nonrebreather mask at 15 lpm you note that she is unresponsive to verbal stimuli, and a quick pinch of the webbing between her fingers results in no response as well. You note that her skin is cold, pale, and diaphoretic, and she has a heart rate of 118, a blood pressure of 122/78, a respiratory rate of 20, and a SaO$_2$ of 99 percent on oxygen. A fingerstick reveals a blood glucose of 28 mg/dL.

You place the patient on the cardiac monitor and attempt to start an 18-g angiocatheter in her right antecubital area without success. You and your partner both take note of the lack of adequate, obvious vasculature on the patient. Rather than making another attempt at intravenous access, you decide to administer glucagon intramuscularly.

While your partner continues to hold the patient's airway open, you assemble your equipment for the glucagon administration. You draw up the diluting solution and mix it with the powder, then draw up the medication into a 3-cc syringe and exchange the 18-g hypodermic needle used to draw the medication for a 1", 22-g hypodermic needle for the medication administration. You take a moment to rethink your plan and confirm *right person, right drug, right dose, right time, right route,* and *right documentation.* You prepare the patient's left deltoid area by swabbing it with an alcohol prep, flatten and stretch the skin over the deltoid muscle, and insert the needle at a 90° angle. You attempt to aspirate for blood without success, then inject the medication over 3 seconds, cover the insertion site with a 2×2 gauze pad, and quickly remove the needle.

In the 8 minutes it takes you to clean up after yourself, put away your equipment, and place the patient on the stretcher, she is able to maintain her own airway and is mumbling incoherently. A fingerstick reveals that her blood glucose has increased to 56 mg/dL. Ask your partner to recheck her vital signs prior to taking her outside to the ambulance for further treatment and transport. ■

CHAPTER 21

Subcutaneous Medication Administration

KEY TERMS

Anaphylaxis

Epinephrine

Hypersensitivity

Hypodermic needle

Intramuscular

Intravenous

Intravenous fluid bolus

Subcutaneous (SQ)

Trendelenburg position

Untoward effects

OBJECTIVES

The student will be able to do the following:

▶ List the indications for the administration of a medication via subcutaneous injection (p. 137).

▶ Describe the proper technique for the administration of a medication via subcutaneous injection (pp. 139–142).

▶ Demonstrate the ability to administer a medication via subcutaneous injection (pp. 139–142).

▶ Value the importance of proper administration of a medication via subcutaneous injection (p. 143).

INTRODUCTION

Subcutaneous (SQ) injection is a method used to place medications under the skin in the fatty area called the subcutaneous layer. The subcutaneous layer lies between the skin and muscle and is composed primarily of loose connective and adipose tissue. It has a minimal vascular supply, resulting in a slow, continuous, sustained absorption into the bloodstream. Medication administered subcutaneously is absorbed at a rate slower than the **intravenous** or **intramuscular** routes, but faster than the oral route.

The injection can be given anywhere there is an area of the skin that can be pinched, though the most common areas for injection are the lateral area of the upper arm over the deltoid muscle, the lateral thigh over the rectus femoris muscle, and the abdomen. Subcutaneous injection sites are shown in red in Figure 21.1. Skin that is easy to pinch contains more subcutaneous tissue that is easier to lift off the underlying muscle, preventing accidental intramuscular injection.

To avoid irritation, infection, and possible abscess formation, subcutaneous injections are usually limited to volumes of 1 mL or less, and are pushed slowly over several seconds. Knowledge of the medication being administered is essential. Knowing the indications, contraindications, adverse reactions, and doses of all medications being administered is important to both avoid and anticipate complications.

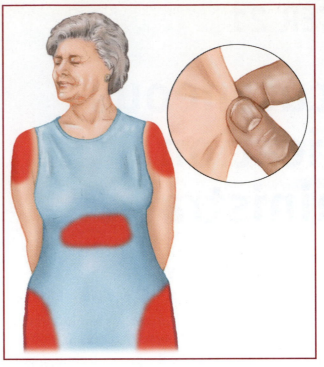

Figure 21.1

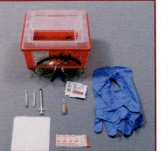

Figure 21.2

EQUIPMENT

You will need the following equipment (Figure 21.2):

- ▶ Gloves
- ▶ Goggles
- ▶ Medication to be administered
- ▶ 1-cc syringe
- ▶ 18-gauge hypodermic needle to withdraw medication
- ▶ 23-gauge, 1" or smaller hypodermic needle for medication administration
- ▶ Alcohol preps
- ▶ 2×2 gauze pads
- ▶ Bandage
- ▶ Sharps container

ASSESSMENT

Use appropriate body substance isolation. Place the patient in a position of comfort and perform an initial assessment, making sure the patient has a patent airway, is breathing adequately, and has a pulse. Obtain level of consciousness and vital signs and perform a focused and detailed assessment. Any life-threatening signs or symptoms should be treated immediately as they are identified.

Subcutaneous medication administration is utilized for a limited number of clinical conditions in the prehospital setting, and may include the administration of **epinephrine** 1:1,000 for asthma or **anaphylaxis** or insulin in cases of hyperglycemia. The assessment of each of these emergencies is much too broad to be included in their entirety in this section, but providers should be familiar with the clinical signs and symptoms associated with all the disease processes that may require a subcutaneous administration of medication.

The desired site for administration should be exposed and free of superficial blood vessels, rashes, swelling, edema, bruises, soreness, and trauma. Adequate peripheral perfusion must be assured prior to subcutaneous administration or the delivered medication may not be sufficiently absorbed into general circulation. If adequate perfusion is not present, an alternative administration route should be considered, such as intravenous or IO administration. If the abdomen will be utilized for a subcutaneous injection, the area around the beltline should be avoided.

Before any medication is administered, confirm *right person, right drug, right dose, right time, right route,* and *right documentation*. Confirm that the patient has no allergies to the medication being administered, and reassess the patient immediately after medication administration for desired and **untoward effects**.

 PROCEDURE: Subcutaneous Medication Administration

1. Take infection control precautions.

   Rationale: It is possible to inadvertently enter a vein when performing a subcutaneous injection, resulting in a splash or spill of blood. Gloves and goggles should be worn during the subcutaneous injection to protect you from a blood-borne pathogen exposure.

2. Explain the procedure to the patient, and confirm that the patient does not have an allergy to the medication being administered.

   Rationale: The subcutaneous injection is going to hurt, with the feeling being similar to a bee sting. Proper planning will minimize the chances of the patient moving or pulling away, causing the injection to have to be repeated. A known allergy to a drug is a contraindication to any medication administration.

3. Confirm the right drug, dose, concentration, and route have been selected for the right patient, and document the information (Figure 21.3).

   Rationale: A mistake with the type of medication, dose of medication, or administration of medication to the wrong patient may at the least under medicate the patient, and in the worst case prove fatal. In addition, some medications can be administered through multiple routes, such as IM, SQ, and IV. However, only one concentration may be appropriate for a certain condition or route of administration.

PEDIATRIC NOTE:

Some medications for pediatric administration, such as epinephrine, not only have a different dose, but a different concentration when administered to children. Be sure to confirm both the concentration and dose when receiving medical control orders for pediatric patients.

4. Assemble the 1-cc syringe and 18-g needle (Figure 21.4).

   Rationale: Many subcutaneous medications will not come in a prefilled syringe, but are often supplied in ampules or vials and must be drawn into a syringe using a **hypodermic needle**.

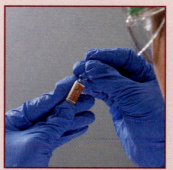

Figure 21.3

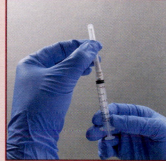

Figure 21.4

continued...

5. Withdraw the proper amount of medication from the ampule or vial into the syringe (see Chapter 17 for the entire procedure) (Figure 21.5).

Rationale: When the medication does not come as a prefilled syringe, it must be drawn into the syringe with a hypodermic needle. Drawing up only the proper amount to be administered can help prevent accidental overdoses since only the desired dose will be in the syringe.

6. Change the hypodermic needle from the one used to draw up the medication to the proper size for subcutaneous injection, usually a size 23 g or smaller (Figure 21.6). Be sure to deposit the used needle in a sharps container.

Rationale: Often, a larger needle (18 g) is used to draw medication into the syringe than is necessary for injection (23–27 g). Additionally, changing needles helps to ensure aseptic technique.

7. Expel any excess air by pointing the syringe to the ceiling and gently pushing excess air out of the needle (Figure 21.7). Be careful not to push an excessive amount of medication out the end of the needle, or your carefully calculated dose will be incorrect.

Rationale: Excess air in the syringe can cause an air embolus in the patient.

8. Reconfirm correct medication, concentration, dose, route of administration, and expiration date.

Rationale: It is possible for medications to be mistaken for another, misplaced by a helper on scene, or for the paramedic to become distracted in the confusion that is typical of the prehospital environment. This second check immediately before the medication is administered is imperative to the prevention of lethal medication errors.

9. Select the appropriate injection site in the subcutaneous tissue of the upper arm over the deltoid muscle.

Rationale: The upper arm of most patients will contain enough fatty tissue for a subcutaneous injection and is easily accessible for the provider.

10. Prepare the injection site by cleaning with an alcohol prep in widening circles from the inside of the injection area to the outside (Figure 21.8).

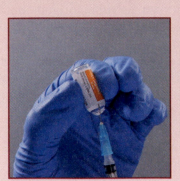
Figure 21.5

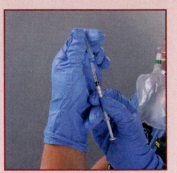
Figure 21.6

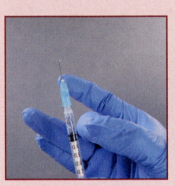
Figure 21.7

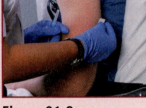
Figure 21.8

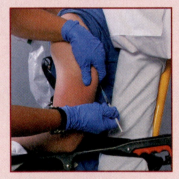
Figure 21.9

Rationale: Using an alcohol prep in widening circles prevents dragging bacteria on the surface of the skin back over the actual injection site.

11. Pinch the skin around the injection site without contaminating the site (Figure 21.9).

Rationale: Pinching the skin helps to gather the subcutaneous layer to avoid deeper penetration into the muscle.

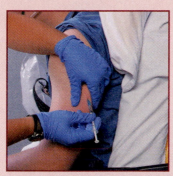

Figure 21.10

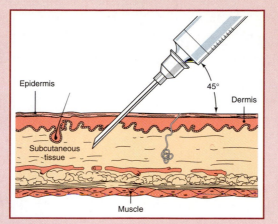

Epidermis

45°

Dermis

Subcutaneous tissue

Muscle

Figure 21.11

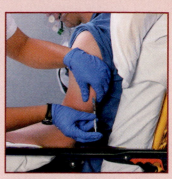

Figure 21.12

> **GERIATRIC NOTE:**
>
> The skin of elderly patients is less elastic, so it may have folds or rolls. Be sure to pinch some fat under all of the skin since the subcutaneous layer has better circulation for medication absorption than does the skin.

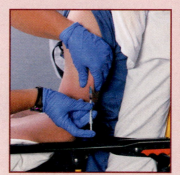

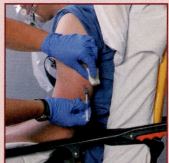

Figure 21.13   **Figure 21.14**

12. Insert the needle quickly at a 45° angle, with the bevel up (Figure 21.10).

    Rationale: This angle of injection helps to deliver the medication to the subcutaneous tissue, rather than the underlying muscle. Medications accidentally given in the muscle will have a different and possibly harmful absorption rate. Additionally, some medications are fat soluble and must be given in the subcutaneous layer or they cannot be absorbed by the body. (See diagram of subcutaneous injection in Figure 21.11.)

13. Aspirate the syringe, confirming that no blood is present in the syringe (Figure 21.12).

    Rationale: Blood in the syringe would indicate that the needle has accidentally been placed in a vein, rather than the subcutaneous tissue. If this occurs, discontinue the procedure and begin again in another location.

14. Inject the medication slowly, over several seconds (Figure 21.13).

    Rationale: Patients can often feel the medication entering the subcutaneous tissue. Administering the medication too quickly can cause unnecessary discomfort.

15. Apply counter-pressure with an alcohol prep or gauze pad, and quickly withdraw the needle (Figure 21.14).

    Rationale: Counter-pressure minimizes discomfort caused by movement of the needle.

16. Apply direct pressure over the injection site with a gauze pad to control any bleeding. Apply a bandage if necessary.

    Rationale: Very minimal bleeding should occur, but is possible. Like any bleeding, it should be controlled with direct pressure and a bandage.

17. Dispose of equipment in an approved sharps container (Figure 21.15).

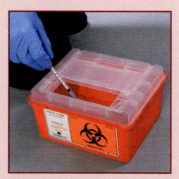

Figure 21.15

continued...

Rationale: The syringe will have a needle attached and must be placed in a sharps container to prevent an accidental needle-stick.

18. Reassess the patient for desired effects of the medication and potentially undesirable side effects (Figure 21.16).

Rationale: Any untoward effects of the medication should be noted and corrected immediately.

19. Document the medication, concentration, dose, time, and effects of the medication on the patient care report.

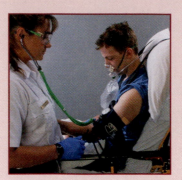

Figure 21.16

ONGOING ASSESSMENT

Reassess the patient before and immediately after administration of any medication. Observe the patient for desired effects of the medication. In some cases, if a single dose of the medication does not produce the desired effects, then a second or subsequent dose may be ordered. Additionally, observe for any undesired effects such as itching, dyspnea, or tachycardia. These effects could indicate an allergy or **hypersensitivity** to the medication. Report these findings to your medical control physician immediately and treat the symptoms present.

Vital signs are an important component of medication administration, and should be measured before and after administration of any medication to determine if the medication had a desirable or undesirable effect on the patient's system. Some medications produce a known drop in blood pressure which might require intervention such as the **Trendelenburg position** or an **intravenous fluid bolus**.

> **GERIATRIC NOTE:**
> Geriatric patients are much more susceptible to changes in blood pressure from medication administration. The circulatory system of older patients does not afford the same ability to vasoconstrict as a compensatory mechanism in response to blood pressure or volume changes. In addition, the elderly commonly have cardiac complications treated with medications such as calcium channel blockers and beta-blockers, resulting in an inability to compensate with increases of heart rate and stroke volume. Therefore, you may observe a more profound drop in blood pressure that may require a change in patient positioning or even a fluid bolus to correct the problem.

▶ PROBLEM SOLVING

► When expelling air from a syringe prior to injection into the patient, be sure not to use too much force which will cause an excessive amount of medication to spill out of the syringe and onto the floor. Not only will this result in a possible underdose of medication to the patient, but some medications are controlled substances; by law, they must have every milligram accounted for.

▶ The procedure described in this chapter utilizes a traditional needle system. However, many systems today are changing to a safety system in which a safety cap is attached to the syringe, allowing the needle to be capped or covered immediately after administration of the medication, helping to prevent accidental needle-sticks.

▶ While not absolutely required, many prehospital systems suggest that patients receiving medication of any kind be connected to a heart monitor prior to and throughout the medication's administration. If a patient is serious enough to require medication therapy in the prehospital setting, he or she is probably ill enough to benefit from cardiac monitoring as well. The monitor can often provide an early warning of an undesirable side effect in addition to other patient signs and symptoms.

CASE STUDY

You are called to a local park where you find a 36-year-old male complaining of shortness of breath and itching in all his extremities. He tells you he was stung 15 minutes ago by a bee. He states that he has a "severe" allergy to bees and that he usually carries an Epi Pen. However, he did not bring his pen to the park today.

He is conscious, slightly pale, and cool to the touch. You note that there is redness and swelling around the area where he was stung. You observe that his respiratory distress is getting worse, and you are starting to hear audible wheezing sounds coming from his airway. His pulse is 136, blood pressure is 94/70, respiratory rate is 28 and labored, and his pulse oximetry is 94 percent on room air. He has wheezing in all lung fields on auscultation.

The patient is placed on oxygen via a nonrebreather mask at 15 lpm. You decide to administer 0.3 mg of 1:1,000 epinephrine subcutaneously to treat the patient's developing allergic reaction. You visualize the upper part of the arm over the deltoid muscle and decide the area is perfect for the subcutaneous injection. As the medication is drawn up you remember from training to check *right person, right drug, right dose, right time, right route,* and *right documentation.* You prepare the injection site by cleaning the area with an alcohol prep, pinch and lift the skin away from the muscle layer underneath, and insert the needle at a 45° angle.

You pull back on the plunger to confirm that you have not entered a vein, then depress the plunger and deliver the medication over a few seconds. The medication is administered without difficulty. You place a 2×2 gauze pad over the injection site, remove the needle from the patient's arm, and dispose of the syringe and needle in a sharps container. A minute after the medication has been injected you and your partner are considering giving a corticosteroid to the patient, when you notice that he is looking, sounding, and feeling better. You immediately reassess to find that the patient's signs and symptoms are almost completely gone. With the approval of the patient, you decide to transport him to the local emergency department. ■

CHAPTER 22

IV Infusion Medication Administration

KEY TERMS

Admixture

Adverse reactions

Buretrol® administration set

Burette

D₅W

Desired effects

Drops per minute

Hypodermic needle

Incompatible

Infiltration

Necrosis

Normal saline

Patent

Piggyback

Primary IV line

Secondary IV line

Unstable

OBJECTIVES

The student will be able to do the following:

▶ List the indications for administration of a medication via IV infusion (p. 144).

▶ Describe the proper technique for administration of a medication via IV infusion to a patient (pp. 145–148).

▶ Value the importance of proper administration of a medication via IV infusion (pp. 145–148).

▶ Demonstrate the ability to administer a medication via IV infusion (p. 150).

INTRODUCTION

Intravenous (IV) infusion is often a preferred method of medication administration, as it provides a high concentration of medication that is rapidly absorbed and distributed, allowing for a rapid onset of action. In addition, medication being administered can be titrated or discontinued according to patient response. In patients with poor perfusion, IV infusion may be the only route of administration by which medications can be readily absorbed.

Establishment of an additional IV line into an existing IV to deliver medication is often referred to as "**piggyback**" administration. This is accomplished by attaching a second IV bag (containing medication) and administration set to an injection port on the existing IV line. The injection port has a small rubber stopper that allows for the insertion of the additional IV tubing to be piggybacked into the port. Medications can be administered continuously over minutes to hours using this technique.

▶ EQUIPMENT

You will need the following equipment (Figure 22.1):

- ► Gloves
- ► Goggles
- ► Alcohol preps
- ► Syringe with needle
- ► 18-gauge hypodermic needle
- ► IV bag
- ► Mini-drip (micro) IV administration set
- ► Tape
- ► Medication label
- ► Patent, previously established primary IV line

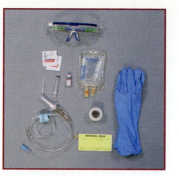

Figure 22.1

ASSESSMENT

Use appropriate body substance isolation. Place the patient in a position of comfort. Perform an initial assessment, making sure the patient has a **patent** airway, is breathing adequately, and has adequate circulation. Obtain level of consciousness and vital signs, and perform a focused or detailed assessment. Any life-threatening signs or symptoms should be treated.

Confirm that the primary IV site is established, patent, and has no **infiltration**. Before any medication is administered confirm *right person, right drug, right dose, right time, right route,* and *right documentation.* Confirm no allergies to the medication to be administered. Reassess the patient immediately after medication administration for **desired** and untoward **effects** of the medication.

PROCEDURE: IV Infusion Medication Administration

1. Take infection control precautions.

   Rationale: Even though the **primary IV line** has been previously established, the piggyback line will still directly access the venous system, creating a potential for exposure to infectious diseases. Gloves and goggles are a must during IV piggyback medication administration.

2. Explain the procedure to the patient (Figure 22.2).

   Rationale: The medication is likely to have noticeable effects or side effects on the patient. Inform the patient about all possible effects of the medication being administered.

3. Select IV fluid appropriate for medication **admixture** (Figure 22.3).

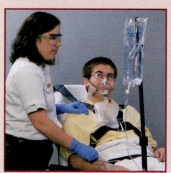

Figure 22.2

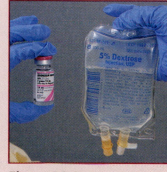

Figure 22.3

continued...

Rationale: Some IV fluids are incompatible with certain medications. As a general rule, **normal saline** or **D_5W** are used for admixture medications.

4. Check the selected IV fluid and packaging for integrity, clarity, and expiration date.

Rationale: All fluid has an expiration date and must not be used if the expiration date has passed. IV fluid that is cloudy or has particulate matter visible in it should be considered contaminated and discarded.

5. Keep in mind the "6 rights" of patients when administering medications. Ensure that you have the:
   ▶ Right patient
   ▶ Right drug
   ▶ Right amount/dose
   ▶ Right route of administration
   ▶ Right time
   ▶ Right documentation

Rationale: Following the "6 rights" ensures that proper safety procedures are used for the administration of any medication. "DICE" is another medication verification used in some systems.

6. Calculate the desired volume of medication needed and, using aseptic technique, draw the desired volume of medication into a syringe. Ensure correct medication, dose, and concentration for the patient (Figure 22.4).

Rationale: By drawing up more medication into the syringe than is needed, you increase the likelihood of an accidental overdose.

7. Using an alcohol prep, clean the medication administration port on the admixture bag (Figure 22.5).

Rationale: Aseptic technique must be used to prevent contamination of the admixture bag.

8. While inverting the IV fluid bag, inject the correct amount of medication into the admixture bag, utilizing the medication injection port (Figure 22.6).

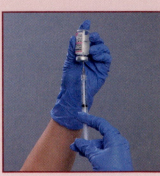
Figure 22.4

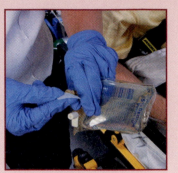
Figure 22.5

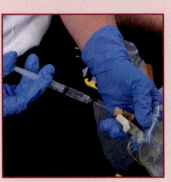
Figure 22.6

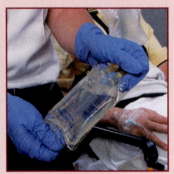
Figure 22.7

Rationale: Depending on the size of the admixture bag, the same amount of medication could double or half the given medication concentration. Successful piggyback medication administration is a combination of proper fluid volume and medication amount to prepare the appropriate medication concentration.

PEDIATRIC NOTE:
Since medication doses for children are so small, check and double-check the math prior to injecting medication into the bag to prevent an overdose.

9. Invert the bag gently several times to mix the medication (Figure 22.7).

Rationale: The medication should be evenly distributed throughout the admixture bag in order to create an admixture and evenly administer the medication over time.

10. Label the admixture bag with the name of the medication, dose, concentration, time and date administered, and your name or initials (Figure 22.8).

    Rationale: Since many medications are infused over hours, a new provider may come on shift during the medication administration and need to know exactly what and how much was administered and is yet to be administered to the patient.

11. Prepare the mini-drip administration set by connecting the tubing to the admixture bag (Figure 22.9), filling the drip chamber, and flushing the tubing, ensuring that no air bubbles remain (Figure 22.10).

    Rationale: Tubing should be purged after the admixture is prepared to ensure that all fluid delivered to the patient contains medication.

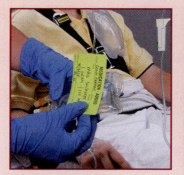

Figure 22.8

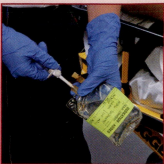

Figure 22.9

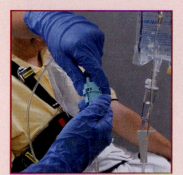

Figure 22.10

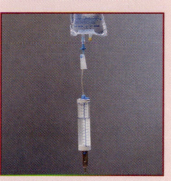

Figure 22.11

> **PEDIATRIC NOTE:**
>
> Special administration sets, called a **Buretrol®** **administration set** (Figure 22.11) or **burette**, may be used for pediatric patients. They contain a special chamber ensuring only the prescribed amount of medication-containing fluid will be administered to patients, preventing a harmful overdose to a pediatric patient.

12. Attach an appropriately sized **hypodermic** **needle** to the administration set. Usually an 18 g or other large needle is used for piggyback medication administration (Figure 22.12).

    Rationale: A large needle ensures that a rapid flow of medication admixture can be infused if appropriate. Smaller needles, such as a 23 g would impede the flow of medication to the patient.

13. Reconfirm allergies to any medications with the patient.

    Rationale: This step should have been completed prior to IV initiation, but the piggyback may be performed by another health care worker. Patient identification and allergies should be reconfirmed by every patient care person prior to administration of any medication.

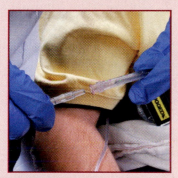

Figure 22.12

> **GERIATRIC NOTE:**
>
> Since the allergen response usually does not occur until the second time someone has been exposed to a medication, younger patients who have not taken or received many medications may not know they are allergic to a particular medication. However, geriatric patients, with their more complicated medical histories, are much more likely to know about their allergies. Be sure they are given ample time to recall the information and relay it to the health care provider.

continued...

14. Cleanse the chosen injection port on the primary IV line with an alcohol prep using an aseptic technique (Figure 22.13).

    Rationale: The port may have been handled by other care providers or otherwise soiled and presents a direct path for infection should any needle puncture the site prior to proper cleaning.

    > **GERIATRIC NOTE:**
    > Similar to transplant patients, or those with liver failure or HIV/AIDS, elderly patients have deteriorating immune systems and are more susceptible to infections that can be life threatening. Take extreme care with aseptic technique to not introduce pathogens into the elderly patient's system.

15. Insert the hypodermic needle attached to the admixture or **secondary IV line** into the injection port of the primary line without contaminating either line (Figure 22.14).

    Rationale: This provides a route of administration for two lines, which will utilize the same existing IV site, eliminating the need for additional painful venipunctures.

16. Stop the flow of the primary line (Figure 22.15).

    Rationale: The primary line, if allowed to continue to flow, will inhibit the flow of the secondary line, making medication administration impossible.

17. Adjust the flow rate of the secondary line consistent with the medication administration order (Figure 22.16).

    Rationale: Failing to set a specific flow rate can result in a medication overdose. All piggyback medications have a rate of administration, such as 30 gtts per minute, or 100 cc per hour.

18. Using tape, secure the piggyback needle into the primary line injection port (Figure 22.17).

    Rationale: This prevents the needle from accidentally being pulled out of the primary line, resulting in the medication running onto the bed or floor instead of into the patient.

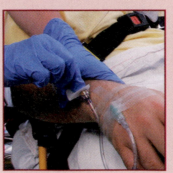

Figure 22.13

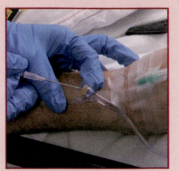

Figure 22.14

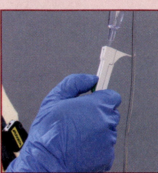

Figure 22.15

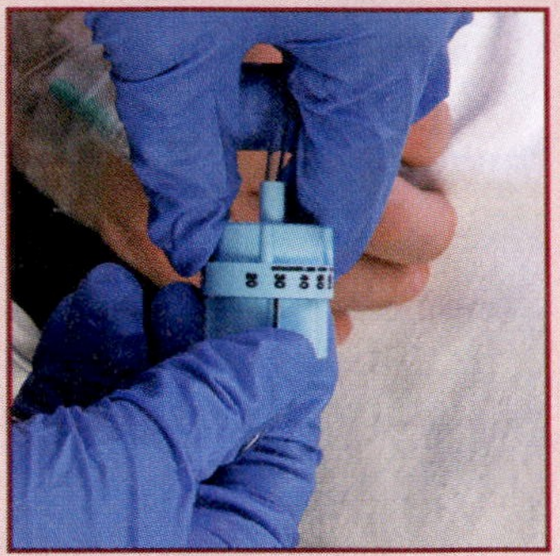

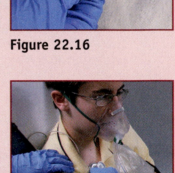

Figure 22.16

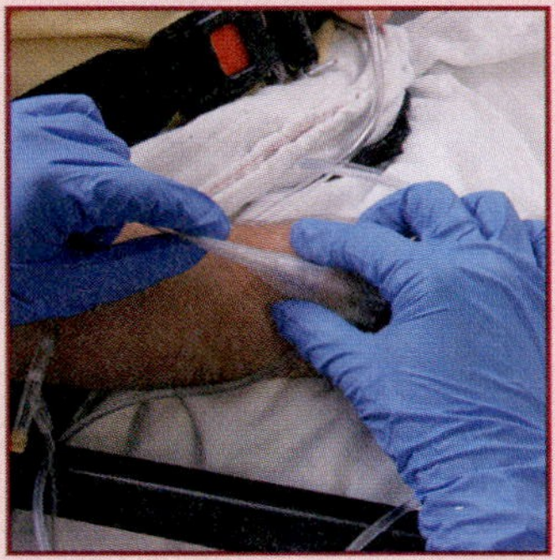

Figure 22.17

Figure 22.18

19. Observe the patient for desired effects of medication and for possible **adverse reactions** (Figure 22.18).

    Rationale: Since the medication is being administered directly into the vein, effects of piggyback medications are usually observable within minutes.

20. Document the medication, concentration, dose, time, and effects of the medication on the patient care report.

ONGOING ASSESSMENT

IV piggyback medication administration requires constant reassessment of not only the secondary piggyback line, but also the primary IV line. Any redness, soreness, swelling, or discoloration at the IV site would indicate that the primary line may be infiltrated and should be discontinued immediately. While it is unsafe to allow infiltration of an IV line when only IV fluid is flowing, it is even more dangerous to allow medications to be infused through a non-patent line. Some medications can cause tissue **necrosis** when infused into an infiltrated IV site.

Administration of any medication can be life-saving as well as life-threatening if not performed properly. All patients who receive medication in the prehospital setting should have serial vital signs performed and most should have continuous cardiac monitoring performed. Most prehospital medications have some effect on the cardiovascular system, and will either affect the heart rhythm or blood pressure. Vital signs should be repeated every 5 minutes for **unstable** patients and every 15 minutes for all other patients. Any adverse reactions, such as lethal dysrhythmias, significant changes in blood pressure, or changes in mental status, would warrant discontinuation of the piggyback administration and contact with medical control immediately. Be sure the receiving facility knows that the patient has had an undesirable reaction to the medication and that it has been discontinued so that they may have an alternative medication available upon arrival to the ED.

▶PROBLEM SOLVING

▶ Some piggyback medications come premixed, such as lidocaine and dopamine. If this is the case, omit steps 3 through 9 of this skill.

▶ Piggyback medication administration requires that a proper flow rate is calculated. Since math can be a weakness of some providers, it is a good idea to get in the habit of working the flow rate calculation by hand, and then double-checking it against either medical control or a prepared drip rate chart available from publishers and pharmaceutical companies.

▶ The piggyback administration set should not be prepared until the medication is already mixed into the admixture bag. Connecting and purging the tubing before injecting the medication into the bag will cause the tubing to be filled with IV fluid only, and no medication. This may result in a delay of onset of medication infusion and action.

▶ While not absolutely required, many prehospital systems suggest that patients receiving medication of any kind be connected to a heart monitor prior to and throughout the administration of the medication. If a patient is serious enough to require medication therapy in the prehospital setting, he is probably ill enough to benefit from cardiac monitoring as well. The monitor can often provide an early warning of an undesirable side effect in addition to other patient signs and symptoms.

▶ Some systems use electric IV pump machines when administering IV piggyback medications. These pumps can be programmed to deliver a specific number of **drops per minute** to ensure a more exact medication dosage is administered to the patient. You must assure you have the proper IV tubing administration set for the machine to be used, as some tubing is **incompatible**.

►CASE STUDY

You arrive at the home of a 63-year-old male complaining of acute onset of substernal chest pain radiating to his neck. During your assessment you note his skin to be pale, cool, and diaphoretic; a pulse of 76 and regular; a blood pressure of 68/40; and respirations of 22 per minute that are shallow and regular. He states that he has a significant history of previous "heart problems" and HTN, and takes many medications.

Based on his PMH, the HPI, and your assessment findings so far, you suspect that the patient is in cardiogenic shock. You place the patient on 100 percent oxygen via a nonrebreather mask at 15 lpm and set up for an IV line while your EMT partner places the patient on the cardiac monitor and prepares the patient for a 12-lead ECG. After the initiation of the IV line, you consider the patient's hypotension and decide against the administration of nitroglycerin, opting for the administration of dopamine at the local medical protocol rate of 10 mcg/kg/minute instead.

As established in protocol, you inject 400 mg of dopamine into a 250-cc bag of normal saline, resulting in a concentration of 1,600 μg/cc. A label is attached to the bag with the amount of dopamine injected, resultant concentration, date, time, and your initials clearly written in indelible ink. A mini-drip IV tubing set is attached to the 250-cc admixture bag, the tubing is purged of air bubbles, and an 18-gauge needle is attached to the administration set. You once again check *right person, right drug, right dose, right time,* and *right route.* You wipe the administration port of your primary IV line with an alcohol prep and insert the needle. You place the piggyback IV line in a mechanical device that regulates the exact flow of medication through the IV tubing. You set the rate on the device to the specific drops per minute based on the dose, patient's weight, and the concentration of the medication. The patient is prepared for transport. You constantly monitor the patient for improvement of his blood pressure and continuously monitor the piggyback drip chamber and delivery device for problems. ■

CHAPTER 23

Medication Administration Using PVAD

KEY TERMS

CVAC—central venous
   access catheter

PICC—peripherally inserted
   central venous catheter

PVAD—preexisting vascular
   access device

OBJECTIVES

The student will be able to do the following:

▶ List the indications for the administration of a medication using a preexisting vascular access device (pp. 151–154).

▶ Describe the importance of proper technique when administrating a medication using a preexisting vascular access device (pp. 151–154).

▶ Describe the proper technique involved in the administration of a medication using a preexisting vascular access device (pp. 155–156).

▶ Demonstrate the ability to properly administer a medication using a preexisting vascular access device (pp. 155–156).

INTRODUCTION

Chances are good that sometime in your EMS career you will provide care to a patient who has a **preexisting vascular access device (PVAD)**, also known as a **central venous access catheter (CVAC)**. These catheters are frequently a source of confusion for paramedics, who commonly question whether a PVAD can be utilized in the prehospital environment. The answer, of course, is yes (providing your protocol allows), but with the caveat that the paramedic needs to be aware of the proper procedures and risks involved.

A PVAD is a catheter inserted into a central vein (central venous catheter, or central line) that permits direct central venous access. Commonly accessed vessels include the cephalic, subclavian, internal and external jugular, and femoral veins. **Peripherally inserted central venous catheters (PICC lines)** are long central catheters placed in a peripheral vessel, commonly the cephalic vein or basilic vein in the bicep or forearm. Central lines and PICC lines are placed percutaneously or by venous cutdown in a controlled, sterile environment, and inserted to a level that places the distal tip in the superior vena cava (SVC) just above the right atrium.

PVADs are inserted in two populations of patients: those requiring dialysis, and those outpatients requiring frequent IV access at home. Outpatient requirements resulting in PICC line placement include the need for

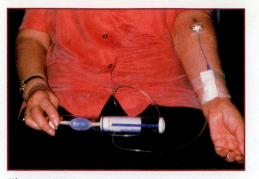

Figure 23.1
Dr. P. Marazzi/Photo Researchers, Inc.

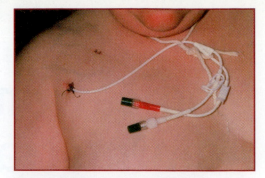

Figure 23.2
Dr. P. Marazzi/Photo Researchers, Inc.

total parenteral nutrition (TPN) and home administration of medication (Figure 23.1) or fluid therapy. In an effort to reduce the number of IV attempts, a PICC line will be placed in patients who require long-term frequent blood draws or medication administration, especially those with poor vasculature or immunosupression.

Examples of PVADs used for dialysis include the Hickman (Figure 23.2), Groshong, and Broviac catheters. Dialysis catheters differ from PICC catheters in that they have larger lumen diameters to allow rapid transfer of large volumes of blood, are tougher to withstand the higher pressures associated with dialysis, and are always impregnated with antibiotics in order to decrease the risk of infection. In addition, they come in single-, double- (Figure 23.3), and triple-lumen variations. The number of lumens any particular catheter has is easy to discern, as the lumens are separated at the distal end.

Each lumen has a colored adapter hub that will have a rubber medication injection port or a needleless injection port and protective cap. Common colors for the adapter hubs include white, blue, red, and brown, with brown always indicating the lumen of largest size. Each lumen of a dialysis catheter has a volume of about 30 mL, and is filled with heparinized saline to prevent blood clotting within the catheter. Simple plastic clamps, located just under the caps, are used to pinch each lumen when not in use to prevent accidental exsanguination.

PICC lines are usually long (16–24 cm), small-diameter, single-lumen, clear polyurethane catheters that exit the bicep or antecubital area (Figure 23.4). The distal end has a hub that attaches to a rubber needle injection port. PICC lines may or may not be impregnated with antibiotics to help reduce the occurrence of infection. Like a dialysis catheter, PICC lines are filled with heparinized saline to prevent the formation of blood clots within the lumen, and have plastic clamps to occlude the lumen when not in use.

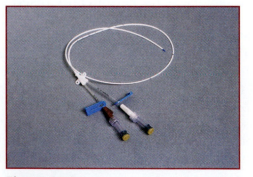

Figure 23.3
Michal Heron

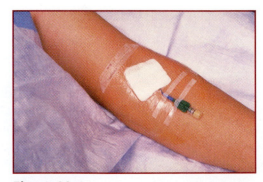

Figure 23.4
Michal Heron

Two indications for use of an existing PVAD are cardiopulmonary arrest and extremis due to circulatory shock, both instances in which peripheral IV attempts may be difficult or impossible. These lines work just like a regular IV line that is established in the prehospital setting. They can be used to administer IV fluids, blood products and medications. The dosages of the medications used are the same as with peripheral IV lines.

While PVADs can be utilized in certain situations, serious complications can arise if the following considerations are not appreciated. First, the heparinized solution must be withdrawn from both dialysis catheters and PICC lines, as "pushing" this solution into central circulation will (especially with the high-volume dialysis catheters) result in interference with coagulation and may have deleterious effects on your patient. You must *always* withdraw 30 cc of blood from a dialysis catheter and 10 cc from a PICC line prior to pushing *anything* forward in the catheter. Inability to withdraw from the catheter is usually a result of occlusion from a blood clot. In such cases, *do not* push saline or medication forward in an effort to "clear" the line, as you will only succeed in introducing a large blood clot directly into the central venous circulation, with a pulmonary embolism being the likely result. The lumen should be promptly recapped and labeled with tape as unusable to prevent accidental use. With a double- or triple-lumen catheter, you can attempt withdrawal from a different lumen.

As a general rule, dialysis catheters should be used only in cases of extreme hemodynamic instability, such as cardiac arrest or shock, as the risk of infection and resultant sepsis increases each time the lumen's protective cap is removed. A patent PICC line can be used for more routine procedures, as its substantially long length decreases the risk of infection, since bacteria have a considerably longer distance to travel. Because of the risk of infection, sterile gloves should be worn when handling uncapped dialysis or PICC lines, and the caps should be swabbed two times with two different alcohol preps prior to access. As with peripheral IV infusion, all air should be removed from IV tubing prior to an infusion being initiated to reduce the risk of air embolism.

In addition to PVADs, a less common form of central venous access is the implantable catheter. Examples of implantable catheters include the Infusaport, Mediport, and Port-A-Cath (Figure 23.5) devices. The device's catheter is placed in the jugular, cephalic, or subclavian vein; its distal end is advanced into the SVC above the right atrium; and the injection port is placed under the skin over a bony prominence such as the sternum or rib. The injection port has a disc-shaped metal body and a self-sealing silicone membrane that allows for multiple needle punctures. A special IV needle, called a Huber needle, is used for access of the device. With special training and access to a Huber needle, these access devices can by utilized be prehospital care providers.

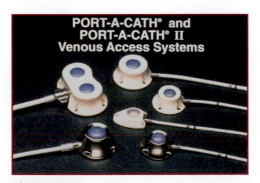

Figure 23.5
SIMS Deltec, Inc.

While you should approach any CVAC device with caution and ensure that you completely understand its function and special considerations prior to use, you should not be afraid of these catheters, as they will save you much-needed time in an emergent situation. In the following example, accessing a PICC line with rubber medication injection port will be illustrated.

▶ EQUIPMENT

You will need the following equipment (Figure 23.6):

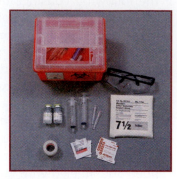

Figure 23.6

- ▶ Sterile gloves
- ▶ Goggles
- ▶ Patent CVAC or PVAD
- ▶ Medication to be administered
- ▶ (2) 18-g hypodermic needle
- ▶ (2) 10-cc syringe
- ▶ Alcohol preps
- ▶ Sharps container
- ▶ Normal saline for flush

ASSESSMENT

Use appropriate body substance isolation. Place the patient in a position of comfort and perform an initial assessment, making sure the patient has a patent airway, is breathing, and has a pulse. Obtain level of consciousness and vital signs and perform a focused and detailed assessment. Any life-threatening signs or symptoms should be treated immediately as they are identified.

PVADs are utilized for a limited number of clinical conditions in the prehospital setting, including cardiac arrest and shock. The absence of a pulse is a straightforward indication that a PVAD can be accessed for use. Patients in shock can be expected to present with tachycardia; tachypnea; hypotension; pale, cold, and diaphoretic skin; anxiety; and an altered mental status. As shock progresses and the patient decompensates, exam findings can progress to bradycardia, bradypnea, developing cyanosis, and loss of consciousness.

Before any medication is administered, confirm *right person, right drug, right dose, right time, right route,* and *right documentation.* Confirm that the patient has no allergies to medication being administered, and reassess the patient immediately after medication administration for desired and untoward effects.

1. Take infection control precautions, including the donning of sterile gloves (Figure 23.7).

   Rationale: Gloves and goggles are required since accessing the PVAD puts the provider in direct contact with the patient's blood and body fluids. In addition, the risk of infection to the patient is significant when accessing these devices.

2. Verify whether or not the patient has any allergies, confirm the medication order, and prepare the appropriate volume of medication (Figure 23.8).

   Rationale: The PVAD should not even be accessed if the patient is allergic to the medication to be administered.

3. Prepare a 10-cc normal saline flush (Figure 23.9).

   Rationale: You will need to flush the catheter with normal saline after the medication administration.

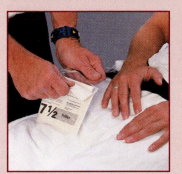

Figure 23.7

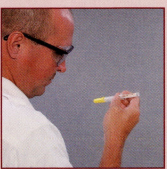

Figure 23.8

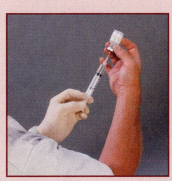

Figure 23.9

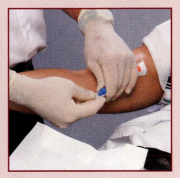

Figure 23.10

> ### PEDIATRIC NOTE:
>
> Even though the pediatric patient is smaller, a 10-cc flush is not excessive. However, in the event you are concerned about fluid overload, a 3- to 5-cc flush can be utilized.

4. Prepare the injection port of a PVAD with an alcohol prep and repeat (Figure 23.10).

   Rationale: The cleansing process is repeated because the risk of infection during prehospital access of a PVAD is so great.

> ### GERIATRIC NOTE:
>
> Remember that geriatric patients have compromised immune systems and are more likely to become seriously ill from bacteria introduced through poor handling of the catheter or port.

5. Unclamp the catheter or port if clamped (Figure 23.11).

   Rationale: You will be unable to aspirate blood or administer medication through the catheter with the clamp secured.

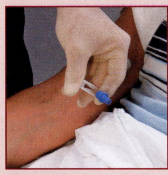

Figure 23.11

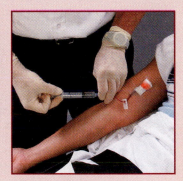

Figure 23.12

6. Attempt to aspirate 10 cc of blood into the syringe (Figure 23.12). If accessing a dialysis catheter, attempt to aspirate 30 cc of blood.

   Rationale: Blood should flow freely into the syringe if the port is free of clots.

continued...

7. After the successful aspiration of blood, administer the desired dose of medication (Figure 23.13) checking to ensure you have the:
   ▶ Right patient
   ▶ Right drug
   ▶ Right amount/dose
   ▶ Right route of administration
   ▶ Right time
   ▶ Right documentation

   Rationale: Only attempt to administer medication after the successful aspiration of blood from the port to prevent dislodging any blood clots from the catheter.

8. Flush the port with 10 cc of normal saline after medication is administered (Figure 23.14). If a dialysis catheter is used, flush with 30 cc of normal saline.

   Rationale: The saline flush will ensure that the medication has reached the bloodstream and is not left in the catheter, port, or tubing.

9. Reclamp the catheter (Figure 23.15).

   Rationale: Clamping the catheter minimizes the chances of leakage or hemorrhage.

10. Dispose of equipment using an approved technique (Figure 23.16).

    Rationale: All needles should be disposed of in a sharps container, and other equipment should be placed in a biohazard bag.

11. Observe the patient for desired effects of medication and for possible adverse reactions.

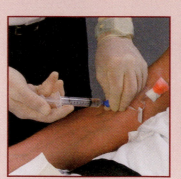
Figure 23.13

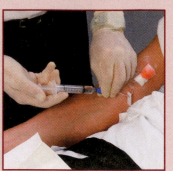
Figure 23.14

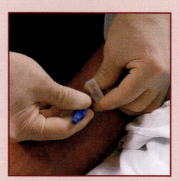
Figure 23.15

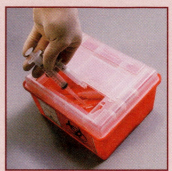
Figure 23.16

Rationale: Since the medication is being administered directly into the vein, effects of piggyback medications are usually observable within minutes.

12. Document the medication, concentration, dose, time, and effects of the medication on the patient care report.

ONGOING ASSESSMENT

Reassess the patient before and immediately after administration of any medication administered through the PVAD. Observe the patient for desired effects of the medication. In some cases, if a single dose of the medication does not produce the desired effects, then a second or subsequent dose may be ordered. Additionally, observe for any undesired effects such as itching, dyspnea, or tachycardia. These effects could indicate an allergy or hypersensitivity to the medication. Report these findings to your medical control physician immediately and treat the symptoms present.

Vital signs are an important consideration, and should be measured before and after administration of any medication to determine if the medication had a desirable or undesirable effect on the patient's system.

▶PROBLEM SOLVING

▶ If administration of volume expanders is anticipated, access the larger, brown port in double- and triple-lumen catheters, if present, as it will be the largest diameter lumen and will allow for the most rapid administration of large volumes of fluid.

▶ If you forget to unclamp the catheter, the saline will not flush easily and you may mistakenly think that the PVAD is not patent.

▶ If you cannot identify the type of PVAD you are looking at, ask the patient or her family. Patients and their family members are often very familiar with the name and use of their PVAD.

▶CASE STUDY

You and your partner have just finished checking your equipment at the beginning of your shift when you are dispatched to a private residence for a cardiac arrest. Upon arrival at the residence, you are led to the patient's bedroom and presented with a 59-year-old female lying supine in bed, pulseless and apneic. You and your partner place the patient on the floor, expose the chest, and notice a Hickman catheter placed in the upper portion of the right chest. Your partner initiates CPR, while you get your monitor ready for a quick look.

After stopping CPR, and performing a quick look, you identify asystole on the monitor and confirm it in two leads. Your partner continues CPR while you intubate the patient, and you have a police officer on scene provide ventilations with a BVM. You attach a macro-drip administration set to a 1,000-cc bag of normal saline and re-move all the air from the tubing, then prepare 1 mg of epinephrine 1:10,000 for ad-ministration.

After donning sterile gloves, you remove the protective cap from the brown port on the Hickman, swab the needleless injection port with two alcohol preps, attach a 30-cc syringe to the port, and are able to aspirate 30 cc of heparinized saline and blood through the catheter. You attach the macro-drip set to the brown Hickman port and run the saline wide open to further ensure catheter patency, pinch the tubing above the medication administration port, and administer 1 mg of epinephrine 1:10,000. You allow the saline to continue to run wide open and continue care ac-cording to your asystole protocol. ■

CHAPTER 24

Rectal Medication Administration

OBJECTIVES

The student will be able to do the following:

▶ List the indications for rectal medication administration
   (pp. 158–159).

▶ Describe the importance of proper administration of a rectal
   medication (pp. 158–159).

▶ Describe the proper technique for performing rectal medication
   administration (pp. 160–162).

▶ Demonstrate the ability to properly perform rectal administration of a
   medication (pp. 160–162).

INTRODUCTION

The rectal administration route takes advantage of the rich vascular supply
of the **rectum**, allowing medications in liquid, gel, or **suppository** form to be
rapidly administered and absorbed in instances when intravenous or
intraosseous cannulation cannot be successfully initiated. In cases of pediatric seizures, the situation probably most commonly encountered by paramedics performing rectal administration of medication in the field, the rectal
route may very well be the most readily available and easily accessible one.

Medications often administered via the rectal route in the acute setting
include diazepam for seizures in pediatric patients, and aspirin for fever in
infants or cardiac emergencies in adults. In addition, sedatives and anti-
emetics are commonly administered via the rectal route. The rectal administration method commonly used by paramedics involves administering a
normal IV dose of medication, such as diazepam, by gently inserting a
needleless 1-cc syringe into the rectum to deposit the medication.

There are three commonly used methods of rectal medication administration; enemas and suppositories in nonacute settings, and the administration of IV-compatible medications in acute settings. An enema is a liquid
bolus injected into the rectum that is absorbed by the rectal mucosa. They
are commonly referred to as small-volume enemas, and come prepackaged
in a squeezable tube with a special tip that is inserted into the rectum. Suppositories are medications molded into a soft, bullet-shaped form that can

easily be slid past the **anus** into the rectum where they dissolve and are readily absorbed by the rectal mucosa.

You will want to make sure that the patient is comfortable, secluded, and covered at all times to assure patient privacy. You also want to make sure that patients are lying on their side with their top thigh flexed so that you can lift the upper buttocks and visualize the rectum. Application of a water-soluble lubricant to the distal end of the syringe will help with ease of insertion into the rectum. Infants can be positioned on their backs, as their natural tendency to roll their pelvis and raise their legs makes the anus easily accessible, and you can hold and raise the legs to expose the anus if needed. After the medication is administered with a syringe, keep patients on their side and hold the buttocks together for 30 to 60 seconds to facilitate retention and absorption. Tell patients not to push or bear down so as not to expel the medication. If delivering a suppository, the buttocks should be held closed for several minutes, and patients kept on their side for 30 minutes.

There are several concerns to be aware of when performing rectal medication administration. One of the most important is to take the hypodermic needle off the syringe prior to inserting the syringe into the rectum. The insertion of a syringe into the rectum often causes **parasympathetic stimulation** via stimulation of the vagus nerve, resulting in bradycardia, so make sure to have the patient attached to a cardiac monitor. You should be particularly careful in administering medications this way to patients who have a cardiac history, as the bradycardia induced by the increased parasympathetic tone may result in profound hypotension and exacerbation of the underlying cardiac disease. Medication should be administered very carefully to patients who complain of abdominal pain.

The rectal route is contraindicated in those patients with recent rectal or prostate surgery, who have diarrhea, who are bleeding from the rectum, or who have any other sign of rectal or anal irritation. One of the disadvantages of rectal administration is incomplete absorption secondary to errors in drug placement, the presence of fecal material, and leakage from the rectum. In addition, inappropriately rough or careless technique can result in anal or rectal trauma, including perforation.

As paramedics most often use the rectal route when treating pediatric patients for seizures, the administration of diazepam to a pediatric patient will be illustrated, though this procedure can easily be adapted for use in patients of all ages and for the administration of suppositories.

▶EQUIPMENT

You will need the following equipment (Figure 24.1):

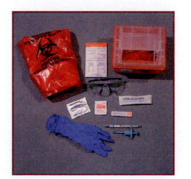

▶ Gloves

▶ Goggles

▶ Medication to be administered

▶ Alcohol prep

▶ Hypodermic needle

▶ 1-cc syringe

▶ Lubricating jelly

▶ Length-based resuscitation tape

▶ Sharps container

▶ Red-bagged receptacle

Figure 24.1

Use appropriate body substance isolation. Place the patient in a position of comfort and perform an initial assessment, making sure the patient has a patent airway, is breathing, and has a pulse. Obtain level of consciousness and vital signs and perform a focused or detailed assessment. Any life-threatening signs or symptoms should be treated immediately as they are identified.

Rectal medication administration is utilized for a limited number of clinical conditions in the prehospital setting, and may include the administration of diazepam for seizures in pediatric and adult patients and aspirin in myocardial infarction. The assessment of each of these emergencies and situations is much too broad to be included in their entirety in this section, but the paramedic should be familiar with the clinical signs and symptoms associated with all the disease processes that may require rectal administration of medication.

The rectum should be inspected and free of irritation, hemorrhoids, active bleeding, or trauma. Assure that there is not a recent history of rectal or prostate surgery or diarrhea. Adequate peripheral perfusion must be assured prior to rectal administration or the delivered medication may not be sufficiently absorbed into general circulation. If adequate perfusion is not present, an alternative administration route should be considered, such as intravenous administration.

Before any medication is administered, confirm *right person, right drug, right dose, right time, right route* and *right documentation*. Confirm that the patient has no allergies to the medication being administered, and reassess the patient immediately after medication administration for desired and untoward effects.

PROCEDURE: Rectal Medication Administration

1. Take infection control precautions.

   Rationale: Gloves and goggles are a must when working around fecal matter that could carry infectious diseases.

2. Confirm drug order with medical control or by using a length-based resuscitation tape (Figure 24.2). Keep in mind the "6 rights" of patients when administering medication. Ensure that you have the:

   ▶ Right patient
   ▶ Right drug
   ▶ Right amount/dose
   ▶ Right route of administration
   ▶ Right time
   ▶ Right documentation

   Rationale: Pediatric drug dosages can vary by one-tenth of a milliliter. Accuracy is imperative to prevent lethal drug overdoses.

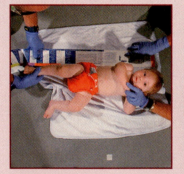

Figure 24.2

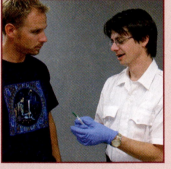

Figure 24.3

3. Verify patient's allergies with a family member or caregiver if possible (Figure 24.3).

   Rationale: Administration of medications to which the patient is allergic can result in a life-threatening anaphylactic reaction. Though a child may not be able to speak for himself, attempt to gather the information about possible allergies from an adult on scene.

4. Select the appropriate medication (Figure 24.4).

   Rationale: Many medications exist in the prehospital drug box. Careful selection of the right drug in the right concentration is crucial to preventing harmful medication administration mistakes.

5. Draw up the correct amount of medication into a 1 to 3-cc syringe (Figure 24.5).

   Rationale: The smallest syringe possible should be used to avoid trauma to the anal and rectal tissue.

6. Remove the needle from the syringe and dispose of it in a sharps container (Figure 24.6).

   Rationale: The needle should not be used during a rectal administration of medication.

7. Lubricate the exterior or syringe tip with a water-soluble lubricating jelly (Figure 24.7).

   Rationale: Lubrication will aid the syringe with entry into the rectum.

8. Place the patient on his side and flex the upper leg forward (Figure 24.8), and spread his buttocks so that the anus is visible (Figure 24.9).

   Rationale: Direct visual contact will be necessary to ensure the syringe is inserted properly into the rectum.

9. Slowly insert the syringe into the rectum, advancing 3 to 5-cm past the rectal sphincter into the rectal canal (Figure 24.10). Do not force if resistance is encountered.

   Rationale: The syringe should be inserted far enough to pass the **anal sphincter** so that medication is absorbed into the rectum itself.

10. Inject medication into the rectum (Figure 24.11).

    Rationale: The medication can be readily absorbed into the vascular rectal tissue.

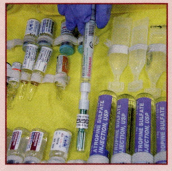

Figure 24.4

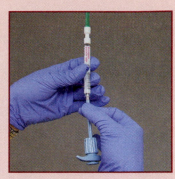

Figure 24.5

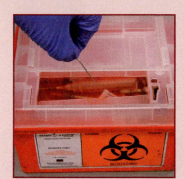

Figure 24.6

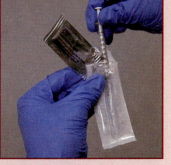

Figure 24.7

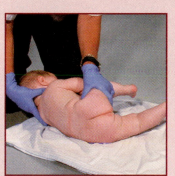

Figure 24.8

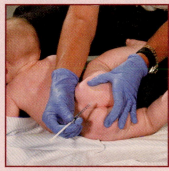

Figure 24.9

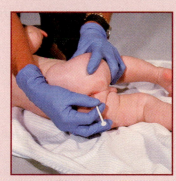

Figure 24.10

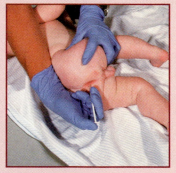

Figure 24.11

continued...

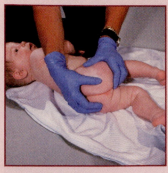

Figure 24.12

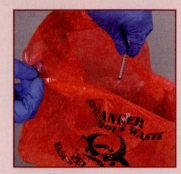

Figure 24.13

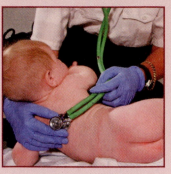

Figure 24.14

11. Slowly withdraw the syringe and press the buttocks together for at least 30 to 60 seconds to facilitate retention of medication in the rectum (Figure 24.12).

Rationale: The medication may leak out if the buttocks remain held open or the patient has a reflexive urge to bear down.

12. Dispose of contaminated equipment in a biohazard bag (Figure 24.13).

Rationale: The syringe will likely be contaminated with a small amount of fecal matter.

13. Closely monitor the airway and breathing status (Figure 24.14).

Rationale: Many medications approved for rectal administration cause respiratory depression.

14. Document the medication, concentration, dose, time, and effects of the medication on the patient care report.

ONGOING ASSESSMENT

Observe the patient immediately after medication administration for desired effects of the medication, as well as adverse or unexpected effects. Manage the symptoms of any adverse effects. For example, administration of diazepam should result in the cessation of seizure activity, but may also depress respirations, necessitating airway control and oxygenation. Additionally, observe for any undesired effects such as itching, dyspnea, or tachycardia, as these effects could indicate an allergy or hypersensitivity to the medication. Report these findings to your medical control physician immediately and treat the symptoms present. In addition, the anal area should be reassessed at some point to assure that there is no hemorrhaging, swelling, irritation, or leakage of medication.

Vital signs should be measured before and after the administration of any medication. Serial vital signs help to establish a pattern of patient improvement or deterioration as a result of the care you provided en route to the hospital. All patients should have at least two sets of vital signs prior to arrival at the hospital.

▶ PROBLEM SOLVING

▶ Valium is a common medication administered rectally to children who are seizing, and is sometimes supplied in packaging that closely resembles morphine and epinephrine. Double- and triple-check that you have selected the correct medication as morphine can cause hypotension and respiratory depression while epinephrine can cause a dangerous tachycardia.

▶ When lubricating the syringe for rectal medication administration, use just enough to ease entry of the syringe into the rectum. Too much lubrication can interfere with the absorption of the medication.

▶ The goal of rectal medication administration is to deposit the medication past the internal and external sphincters and into the rectal canal. A 1-cc syringe is sufficient to accomplish this in an infant, but a feeding tube attached to the end of the syringe may be necessary in older children and adults to reach the desired location.

▶ To administer a suppository, warm the suppository in your gloved hand or run it under warm water to begin dissolving the pellet, lubricate your insertion finger with water-soluble lubricant, and insert the suppository into the rectal canal with your lubricated finger.

▶CASE STUDY

You and your partner are dispatched to a private residence for a pediatric seizure. When you approach the house, the father meets you at the door and states that his 4-month-old daughter has been seizing for approximately 3 minutes without stopping. You ascertain her history from the father and gather that the child has not been sick in the recent weeks and has received all the inoculations typical for a child her age. When you walk into the child's room, you see a young girl lying on the bed seizing, and you note the presence of central cyanosis. You immediately have your partner get out a nonrebreather oxygen mask to provide high-flow oxygen.

You call base to get a standing order for valium. You receive the order, but you are unable to start an IV. Your protocol does not allow you to start IOs, so you advise the parents of the procedure you are to perform, and get the child ready for rectal medication administration. You place the child on her side, draw up the appropriate amount of medication into the syringe, and get out some KY lubricating jelly. You apply KY to the tip of the syringe, lift the upper buttocks, visualize the rectum, insert the syringe, and administer the medication. You squeeze the buttocks together, and package the child for transport to the local hospital for further care. ■

CHAPTER 25

Use of Length-Based Resuscitation Tape

OBJECTIVES

The student will be able to do the following:

▶ List the indications for use of a length-based resuscitation tape (pp. 164–165).

▶ Value the importance of using a length-based resuscitation tape when indicated (pp. 164–165).

▶ Describe the proper technique for use of a length-based resuscitation tape (pp. 165–166)

▶ Demonstrate the ability to use a length-based resuscitation tape (pp. 165–166).

INTRODUCTION

Length-based **resuscitation tape** is used to assist the health care professional in estimating patient body weight and determining proper medication doses and equipment sizes. One of the more widely used resuscitation tapes is the **Broselow® tape** (Figure 25.1). This tool is very helpful in stressful situations, when drugs, dosages, and equipment sizes may have slipped your mind. The tape is utilized by placing it alongside the patient and noting patient length against the tape. An estimate of weight based on length is offered on the tape, and the corresponding area on the tape lists appropriate drug doses and infusion rates based on the estimated weight. In addition, the infant matches up with a "**color zone**" on the tape. Appropriately sized equipment that has been prepared and arranged in a corre-

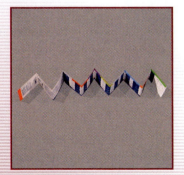

Figure 25.1

sponding colored pouch can then be retrieved, allowing for rapid assembling of the correct sized equipment required for resuscitation. If equipment has not been prepared ahead of time, the resuscitation tape lists the appropriate sizes for equipment such as the oral airway, bag-valve mask, oxygen mask, laryngoscope blade, and endotracheal tube, which must then be assembled by the rescuer.

This rainbow-colored device is very easy to apply and painless to the pediatric patient.

The tape is laminated so that it can be easily cleaned. In some EMS communities, it is protocol to use the Broselow® tape on every pediatric patient.

▶ EQUIPMENT

You will need the following equipment (Figure 25.2):

▶ Gloves
▶ Goggles
▶ Length-based resuscitation tape

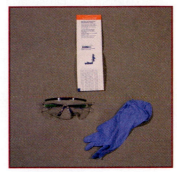

Figure 25.2

ASSESSMENT

Use appropriate body substance isolation precautions. Place the child in the supine position. Perform an initial assessment, making sure the patient has a patent airway, is breathing, and has adequate circulation. If there are any issues with the ABCs that will need to be addressed, a length-based resuscitation tape should be utilized immediately to aid in equipment selection, medication dose determination, and appropriate fluid volume administration. Vital signs should be obtained and a focused and detailed assessment may need to be performed. Any life-threatening signs or symptoms should be treated immediately, and the patient should be reassessed continuously.

PROCEDURE: Use of Length-Based Resuscitation Tape

1. Take infection control precautions.

   Rationale: Gloves and goggles are standard equipment when working with any patient in the prehospital setting.

2. Place the patient in the supine position.

   Rationale: Many patients will not be able to stand alone, and an accurate measurement cannot be obtained when a parent or caregiver is holding the child.

3. Place the tape next to the patient so that the multicolored side is facing up and the red end, displaying the words "measure from this end," is even with the top of the patient's head (Figure 25.3).

   Rationale: The top of the head will be the starting point for the measurement.

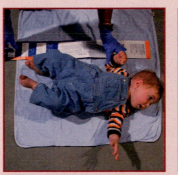

Figure 25.3

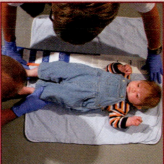

Figure 25.4

4. Holding the red end in place, straighten the tape along the length of the patient, assuring that the infant is not in a flexed position (Figure 25.4).

continued...

PROCEDURE: Use of Length-Based Resuscitation Tape
(continued)

Rationale: Any folds in the tape or flexing in the patient may cause an inaccurate reading, resulting in the wrong medication dosage.

5. Note and document the color or letter block and weight range for the patient (Figure 25.5).

    Rationale: The color block identifies the proper size of equipment to be used for this patient while the weight ranges are used to calculate proper medication dosages.

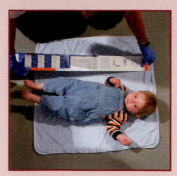

Figure 25.5

ONGOING ASSESSMENT

Once the patient has been properly measured using the length-based resuscitation tape, further measurements will not be necessary. However, frequent reassessment of the patient's condition is required. Vital signs should be measured every 5 minutes for unstable patients, and every 15 minutes for stable patients. At least two sets of vitals should be taken on every patient prior to arrival at the ED.

▶ PROBLEM SOLVING

▶ Infants tend to lie in a flexed position. Be sure to manually straighten their legs before taking their measurement on the resuscitation tape since the total premise of the tape is based on the length of the patient. Failure to do so will cause a "too small" reading and inaccurate medication dosages to be given.

▶ Obvious deviations from the standard size child such as obese children should be considered when providing weight-based medications. If a child is larger than the resuscitation tape, then appropriate adult dosages and equipment are usually utilized based on weight, rather than length. A parent or caregiver on scene may know the child's actual weight.

▶ If a child is indeed standing, and his condition does not warrant placing him in the supine position, then the tape is used in reverse of the standard method. Place the red arrow at his feet, and extend the tape upward, noting the color and weight range at the top of his head (Figure 25.6).

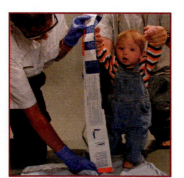

Figure 25.6

▶ CASE STUDY

You are called to the home of an affluent celebrity for a full arrest. When you arrive on scene and encounter a female in her 40s at the front door, you ask "Where is the patient?" She responds frantically, "My baby is blue." Your heart starts to race, because you had no idea that this was going to be a pediatric full arrest. You try and think of drugs and dosages as the mother leads you to the back of the house into the laundry room. As you approach the patient, you see a 3-year-old girl lying supine on the floor of the laundry room.

You rule out the need for c-spine precautions, and realize that the child is unresponsive, apneic, and pulseless. You ask your partner to start CPR while you get the monitor ready. You hook the child up to the monitor and note asystole. You confirm asystole in two leads while your partner begins airway management. You pull out the Broselow® tape and size up the child to be in the purple zone. You read the chart and see that epinephrine 1:10,000, 0.11 mg or 1.1 mL, is your first dose. You establish an IV and administer the first dose of epinephrine. With the airway managed and the first drug on board, you rapidly prepare for transport to the hospital following local protocol for pediatric arrest in asystole. ■

CHAPTER 26

Intraosseous Infusion

KEY TERMS

Bone marrow

Broselow® tape

Buretrol® administration
   set

Caudad

Epiphyseal plate

Infiltration

Sternum

Tibia

Trocar

Venous plexus

OBJECTIVES

The student will be able to do the following:

▶ List the indications for performing intraosseous access and infusion (pp. 168–171).

▶ Describe the importance of properly performing intraosseous infusion (pp. 168–171).

▶ Describe the proper technique used in performing intraosseous access and infusion (pp. 171–174).

▶ Demonstrate the ability to perform intraosseous access and infusion properly (pp. 171–174).

INTRODUCTION

Historically, intraosseous (IO) access was a procedure reserved for pediatric patients when intravenous (IV) access proved impossible. New science and technology advancements have demonstrated this procedure to be both safe and effective for patients of any age. Intraossesous (IO) access is now second to IV access as a preferred route for both fluid and medication administration. Because absorption of medications given via the ET tube route is poor and it is difficult to establish a correct ETT dose, IO is the preferred route over ETT administration. Intraosseous (IO) medication dosing is the same for all medications given the IV route. Introsseous (IO) access has proven to be a safe effective method for fluid resuscitation, medication administration, and laboratory evaluation in both the pediatric and adult patient.

Intraosseous (IO) access involves the placement of a rigid needle into the noncollapsable **venous plexus** in the **bone marrow.** This allows for the rapid and reliable administration of medications, fluids, and blood products when peripheral intravenous access cannot be established. IO access can usually be accomplished quickly (within 30–60 seconds), and allows for rapid absorption of medications into central circulation. Onset of action and drug levels of medication administered via the IO route are comparable to those administered intravenously.

Indications for IO access and infusion include the presence of cardiac arrest or shock, unresponsiveness, and unsuccessful attempts at peripheral IV access. In cases of cardiac arrest and shock, peripheral IV access will be difficult due to flaccid vasculature, and IO access should be considered a first-line intravenous option. Remember that IO access is reserved for those critical patients who are severely hemodynamically compromised and require aggressive care that necessitates venous access. It is not an access route to consider in stable patients.

Contraindications for IO access include fractures to the pelvis or a bone located proximal to the insertion site, and a fracture or previous IO attempt in the bone considered for access. Relative contraindications to IO insertion include cellulitis or other infection, burns, or soft-tissue injury at the insertion site. In addition, an age of 6 has been commonly cited as a cutoff for use of the proximal tibia as an insertion site due to the difficulty of manually inserting a needle into the more developed, thicker bone typical of older patients. However, as newer technology is developed, the **tibia** is being used as the insertion site for all ages.

A typical IO needle consists of a handle, a body with an adjustable plastic disk, a 14 to 18 gauge needle, and a removable **trocar** to support the needle during insertion and prevent occlusion with tissue or bone (Figure 26.1). Specific products, made for sternal placement and high density bone placement are now available to expedite IO placement in both adult and pediatric patients.

Intraosseous access can be established in many sites. The proximal tibia is the most common location for IO placement in both adults and children. The distal tibia, just above the medial malleolus, the distal femur, the anterior-superior iliac spine are other acceptable locations. In older children and adults the **sternum,** distal tibia, and distal ulna may be used for IO insertion. Adults IOs can be initiated anywhere bone marrow is accessible, and numerous methods of achieving access have been developed and are available, including small hand-held electric drills and spring or pneumatic powered IO "guns." Any of these methods are acceptable and are gaining popularity for field use.

To establish IO access in the proximal tibia (Figure 26.2), position the patient's leg with a rolled towel to provide slight flexion and external rotation. Clean the insertion area with a disinfectant agent such as alcohol preps and betadine solution. Stabilize the leg with one hand while the inserting the IO needle through the skin over the flat anteromedial surface of the tibia (Figure 26.2), with the other hand. This area is located about two finger widths below the tibial tuberosity.

While holding the needle at 90° to the bone surface (or slightly **caudad,** to avoid the **epiphyseal plate**), a firm twisting motion is used to advance the needle through

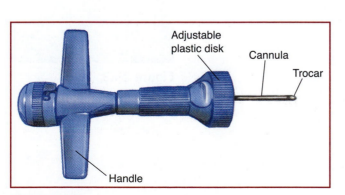

Adjustable plastic disk
Cannula
Trocar
Handle

Figure 26.1

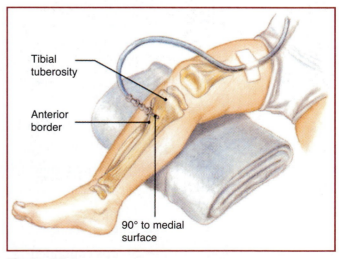

Tibial tuberosity
Anterior border
90° to medial surface

Figure 26.2

the bone and into the marrow cavity. A "popping" sensation and a sudden decrease in resistance will indicate entrance into the marrow cavity. While stabilizing the IO with your hand, unscrew the cap and remove the trocar from the body of the IO needle. You should then attempt to aspirate bone marrow, which may or may not prove successful even with proper entry into the marrow cavity. If you think that you are in the marrow cavity, carefully attempt to flush 5 cc of saline through the IO and immediately observe for swelling at the insertion site. If the flush injection is unsuccessful and infiltration is observed in the surrounding tissues, remove the needle and attempt the procedure in another bone. If the IO flushes freely and no swelling is observed, stabilize the device by lowering the adjustable plastic disk to the skin surface, then remove the flush syringe and attach a prepared IV bag and administration tubing. Further stabilization of the IO needle can be accomplished by using bulky dressings to support the IO and taping them in place, much as you would secure a penetrating object. Roller gauze or Kling® is commonly used for this purpose.

Any medication that can be administered through an IV access site can be administered through an IO. In addition, venous blood for blood chemistry determination, blood gas analysis (BGA), and type- and cross-matching can be obtained from the IO. Administration of sodium bicarbonate through the IO, however, can affect BGA, rendering results of samples withdrawn from the IO questionable. In addition, all crystalloids, colloids, and blood products can be administered as well.

The onset of action of medication and blood medication levels are comparable for IV and IO routes of administration. Medications administered through the IO route, should be flushed with 5–10 mL of normal saline to facilitate delivery to central circulation. An infusion pump and pressure bag or forceful manual pressure may be needed for rapid volume infusion of viscous drugs, fluid solutions or blood.

Complications associated with IO can occur and include fractures, **infiltration** of fluid into tissues, pulmonary embolism from fat or bone marrow absorbed into the circulatory system, local infections, and damage to the growth plate and joints. Careful technique and attention to detail can reduce the rate of occurrence of many of these complications. To rule out the possibility of misplacement or extravasation, the entire circumference of the limb around the insertion site should be inspected and palpated for swelling, bleeding, or any other signs of infiltration.

▶EQUIPMENT

You will need the following equipment (Figure 26.3):

▶ Gloves

▶ Goggles

▶ Towel

▶ IV fluid

▶ Administration set

▶ IO needle

▶ Three-way stopcock

▶ 5-cc syringe

▶ 18-g hypodermic needle

▶ Alcohol preps

▶ 1″ tape

▶ Bulky dressing such as roller gauze or Kling®

▶ Sharps container

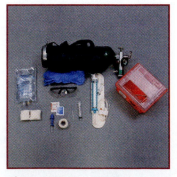

Figure 26.3

ASSESSMENT

Use appropriate body substance isolation. Place the patient in a position of comfort. Perform an initial assessment, making sure the patient has a patent airway and circulation. Obtain level of consciousness and vital signs, and perform a focused or detailed assessment. Any life-threatening signs or symptoms should be treated.

Any patient who is in cardiac arrest, evidenced by pulselessness and apnea, is an immediate candidate for IO access. In addition, patients in shock presenting with profound hypotension; altered mental status; decreased level of consciousness; cold, pale, or cyanotic skin; and flaccid vasculature should have an IO placed immediately if IV attempts prove unsuccessful. In such a situation, where venous access is required quickly for rapid, aggressive resuscitation, attempts at peripheral IV access may take more time and have a lower success rate than IO access. Inspect the limb to be accessed and pelvis to ensure that there are no fractures and that no previous IO attempts are noted. Ideally, the area will also be free of rashes, swelling, edema, bruises, and soreness. To demonstrate the procedure of IO access, the insertion of a handheld IO needle into a pediatric patient will be illustrated.

PROCEDURE: Intraosseous Infusion

1. Take infection control precautions.

   Rationale: The IO procedure will expose the rescuer to blood and bone marrow, both of which carry potentially infectious material. Gloves and goggles are a must during IO insertion.

   ### PEDIATRIC NOTE:

   Special administration sets, often called a **Buretrol®** (Figure 26.4) **administration set** or burette, may be used for pediatric patients. They contain a special chamber ensuring only the prescribed amount of fluid will be administered, preventing fluid overload in pediatric patients.

2. Check the selected IV fluid and packaging for integrity, clarity, and expiration date (Figure 26.5).

   Rationale: All fluid has an expiration date and must not be used if the expiration date has passed. IV fluid that is cloudy or has particulate matter visible in it should be considered contaminated and discarded.

3. Prepare the administration set by connecting tubing to the IV fluid bag, filling the drip chamber, flushing the administration set and

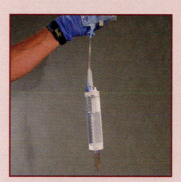 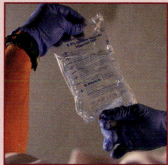

Figure 26.4   Figure 26.5

   extension tubing with fluid, and ensuring that no air bubbles remain in the line.

   Rationale: Air bubbles in the tubing could put the patient at risk for an embolism.

   ### GERIATRIC NOTE:

   Geriatric patients are especially susceptible to embolisms due to comorbidities and lowered cardiovascular reserve.

4. Prepare a saline flush by attaching a hypodermic needle to a syringe and drawing 5-10 mL of

   continued...

normal saline into the syringe from the IV bag. Be sure to cleanse the port of the IV bag with alcohol prior to puncturing the port with the needle (Figure 26.6).

Rationale: The saline flush will be used to confirm needle placement in the marrow cavity.

5. Tear the tape and prepare the padding for securing the IO needle after the puncture (Figure 26.7).

Rationale: A commercial securing device does not yet exist for IO needles. Tape and padding is still the preferred method of securing the device and preventing the needle from being dislodged.

6. Identify proper anatomical landmarks for IO puncture. The most common location is the flat area two finger-widths (or 1–3 cm) below the tibial tuberosity on the medial side of the leg (Figure 26.8).

Rationale: This location is flat, has the least amount of soft tissue to penetrate, and is also well below the growth plate, minimizing the risk of any permanent damage from the puncture.

 GERIATRIC NOTE:

Some IO protocols allow penetration of the sternum, instead of the tibia, for adult or geriatric IO placement. Check your local protocol to see if this option exists for your geriatric patients.

7. Place a rolled towel under the patient's leg, and stabilize the leg without placing your hand behind the puncture site (Figure 26.9).

Rationale: Stabilizing the patient's leg prevents it from moving during the puncture and interfering with the attempt. Not placing your hand behind the puncture site decreases the risk of accidental needle-stick.

8. Cleanse the IV site with alcohol and/or betadine using an aseptic technique (Figure 26.10).

Rationale: Aseptic technique decreases the risk of infection.

9. Perform the IO puncture using a firm but controlled twisting or screwing motion until a

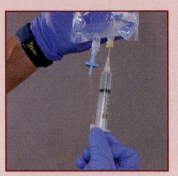

Figure 26.6

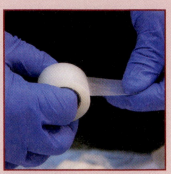

Figure 26.7

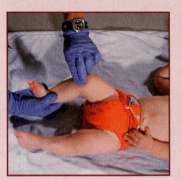

Figure 26.8

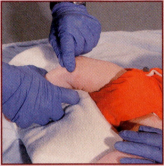

Figure 26.9

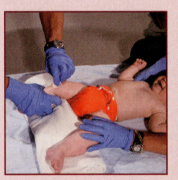

Figure 26.10

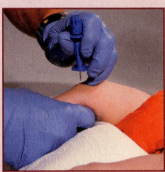

Figure 26.11

popping sensation or sudden decrease in resistance is felt. This is how you know you are now in the marrow. The needle should be at a 90° angle to the tibia or slightly caudad (Figure 26.11).

Rationale: The twisting motion helps to introduce the needle without splintering or fracturing of the bone, and inserting the needle at 90° or slightly caudad prevents insult to the joint or epiphyseal plate.

PEDIATRIC NOTE:

Since children are still growing, take care to avoid the growth plate during your IO puncture. Interruption in this growth area could cause permanent growth damage, resulting in one leg being shorter than the other.

10. Unscrew the cap on the IO needle and remove the trocar (Figure 26.12).

    Rationale: Removing the trocar will allow you to attach the syringe, aspirate for bone marrow, and attempt to flush the IO.

11. Dispose of the trocar in a sharps container (Figure 26.13).

    Rationale: The IO trocar should be treated like any other needle and disposed of properly.

12. Attach the syringe to the IO needle and attempt to aspirate bone marrow (Figure 26.14).

    Rationale: Aspiration of marrow is a positive indication that the needle has entered the bone marrow cavity. If no marrow is aspirated, the IO may still be in the proper location, but it is yet to be determined.

13. Slowly inject the saline flush while feeling for resistance and observing for swelling around the entire circumference of the limb (Figure 26.15).

    Rationale: Resistance or swelling indicates a failed attempt. If resistance is met or swelling noted, attempts at flushing should be immediately suspended and the IO removed, even if marrow was initially aspirated.

14. Connect the administration set to the catheter and run IV fluid for a brief period to further confirm patency of the IO line (Figure 26.16).

    Rationale: The fluid should flow freely if the line is patent. If the fluid does not flow freely, consider discontinuing use of the IO line.

15. Adjust the flow rate as appropriate for the patient's condition (Figure 26.17).

    Rationale: Failing to set a specific flow rate can result in fluid overload, a dangerous patient complication.

16. Lower the adjustable plastic disk to the skin to secure the needle (Figure 26.18).

    Rationale: Securing the needle decreases the risk of dislodgement.

17. Secure the needle with tape and a bulky dressing (Figure 26.19).

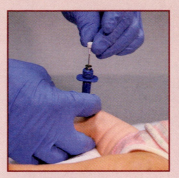

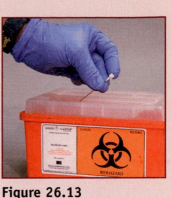

Figure 26.12   **Figure 26.13**

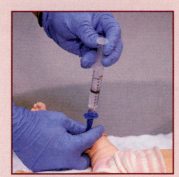

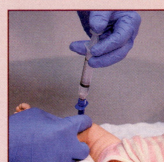

Figure 26.14   **Figure 26.15**

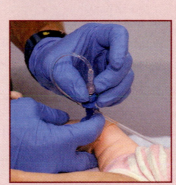

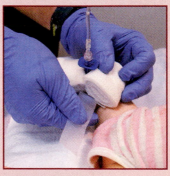

Figure 26.16   **Figure 26.17**

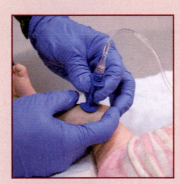

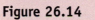

Figure 26.18   **Figure 26.19**

Rationale: Securing the needle further with roller gauze or Kling® provides additional protection against catheter dislodgement.

continued...

18. Reassess the patients for desired effects of the medication and potentially undesirable side effects.

Rationale: Any untoward effects of the medication should be noted and corrected immediately.

19. Document the medicaiton, concentration, dose, time, and effects of the medication on the patient care report.

ONGOING ASSESSMENT

Intraosseous infusion is rarely the first choice for IV access. IO is used when peripheral sites are unobtainable. Usually, an IV is unobtainable only when the patient is poorly perfusing, which by definition makes the patient with an IO in place a critical or unstable patient. Vital signs on these patients, including pulse, respirations, and blood pressure, should be measured at least every 5 minutes. Serial vital signs should be available upon arrival at the hospital to demonstrate to ED staff that the patient has had a trend of improvement or deterioration during the time you have cared for him.

The same fluids and medications, including blood products, can then be administered through a peripheral or central line, as well as through the IO line. However, just like those lines, the IO is subject to complications such as occlusion and dislodgement. Pay careful attention to the patency of the line. If fluid or medications become difficult to infuse through the line, or if redness, swelling, pain, or a hematoma develops at the IO puncture site, discontinue the line immediately. Remember to look for signs of extravasation on the posterior part of the leg as well as the anterior.

▶ PROBLEM SOLVING

▶ When stabilizing the patient's leg for IO puncture, avoid the temptation to hold under the calf muscle or under the knee. Position your nondominate hand above or below the puncture site to minimize the risk of the needle penetrating the entire tibia and entering your hand when placed underneath.

▶ It is not uncommon to fail to get marrow when aspirating after the IO puncture, and lack of marrow aspirate may or may not indicate a failed attempt. The ease of the flush is usually a better indicator of patency.

▶ If you meet resistance when you attempt to flush, try withdrawing the IO needle slightly, then reattempt the flush. The needle may be impaled in the posterior wall of the marrow cavity and the needle lumen occluded. Freeing the needle tip from the posterior wall may unobstruct the needle and allow adequate flow.

▶ Since a bulky dressing is used to secure the IO needle, IV fluid can sometimes be absorbed into the dressing when the IO needle is dislodged and extravasation with leakage is occuring. Be sure to examine the dressing for absorption of fluid periodically during transport as part of your ongoing assessment to ensure that the IO remains properly placed.

►CASE STUDY

You and your partner are backing your ambulance into the station when you are dispatched to an unconscious infant. While responding, the dispatcher informs you that the first-responding engine company on scene has reported that the patient is in cardiac arrest and CPR is in progress. You arrive on scene and find the firefighters in the living room with the patient, providing CPR and ventilations. Your partner prepares the intubation equipment as you place the patient on your cardiac monitor and confirm asystole in two leads. You take a quick look for an acceptable IV site, don't identify one, and decide that an IO insertion is your best bet at this point for rapid venous cannulation.

You attach an administration set to a 500-cc bag of normal saline and flush the line. You then draw up 5–10 cc of saline into a 10-cc syringe for a flush. You tear some tape and open two rolls of Kling® to secure your IO. You prop the patient's leg up on a towel, and have a firefighter hold the leg steady at the ankle as you identify the flat anteromedial surface about 2 cm below the tibial tuberosity and cleanse the site with an alcohol prep. Holding the needle slightly caudad at the insertion site, you use a screwing motion while providing firm, controlled pressure to insert the needle, and quickly feel a pop and a decrease of resistance indicating that you are in the marrow cavity.

After removing the trocar, you attach the 5-cc syringe and fail to aspirate any marrow, but the IO flushes easily without any resistance or swelling to the anterior or posterior leg. You remove the syringe and attach the IV tubing to the IO, assure that it still flows freely, then adjust the securing disk against the skin. Finally, you secure the IO as you would an impaled object, with Kling® wrapped around the base and held in place with tape. As you finish securing the IO, your partner is sizing the patient with **Broselow® tape** to determine the correct epi dose to administer IO. ■

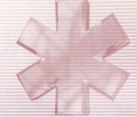

SECTION 3

CARDIAC MANAGEMENT SKILLS

In terms of cardiac arrest management, the ambulance is a mobile emergency department. In fact, new guidelines for cardiac care suggest that the patient 's best chance of resusitation is when he is managed in the prehospital setting as few, if any, treatments or procedures are available in the emergency department that are not available to the patient via EMS.

EMS provides not just treatment via pacing and defibrillation, but monitoring of the cardiac rhythm as well. Cardiac monitoring can be an important diagnostic tool both for primary cardiac conditions, as well as side effects of other treatments and medications administered by the ALS provider. By monitoring the cardiac rhythm you can tell if your intubation attempts are causing a dangerous bradycardia, or if the morphine you administered for a femur fracture is causing cardiovascular side effects. Prehospital 12-lead ECG is responsible for reduced door-to-drug and door-to-cath lab times of up to 1 hour, saving precious heart muscle and returning patients to a quality of life not previously possible.

Your ability to care for your patient using cardiac skills will be a direct result of your diligence in learning the different rhythms and dysrhythmias. You should be practicing not only on static rhythm strips, but also in the dynamic arena of real patient care situations where you have both patient and ambulance movement interfering with what you wish could be a perfect rhythm strip.

CHAPTER 27

Application of Cardiac Monitor

KEY TERMS

Artifact

Diaphoresis

Electrodes

Leads

Limb leads

MCL$_1$

OBJECTIVES

The student will be able to do the following:

▶ List the indications for the application of a cardiac monitor (pp. 178–179).

▶ Describe the importance of proper application of a cardiac monitor (pp. 178–179).

▶ Describe the proper technique for the application of a cardiac monitor (pp. 180–181).

▶ Demonstrate the ability to apply a cardiac monitor (pp. 180–181).

INTRODUCTION

A cardiac monitor should be applied anytime ALS interventions are to be performed. The monitor allows you to identify the patient's heart rhythm, rate, and any electrical abnormalities. However, the presence of electrical activity on the oscilloscope of a cardiac monitor does not give the paramedic any information as to the pumping efficacy of the heart. As such, you must confirm that the rate and rhythm on the monitor correlates with a pulse and adequate blood pressure.

Electrodes, consisting of an adhesive pad with a conductive substance in the center, are designed to be applied to the **leads** (also referred to as monitoring cables, or wires), and then placed on the patient's limbs. The term Lead, when capitalized is used to describe the monitoring and recording of electrical activity between two electrodes. Lead II, for example, records the electrical activity between electrodes placed on the left leg and right arm. Depending on what part of the heart is being viewed, or how many views of the heart are desired, as few as 3 leads, or as many as 15 leads, can be used.

The 3-lead or 4-lead system is the standard EMS monitoring system and the 12-lead is typically used to rule out myocardial infarction. In a standard 3-lead application, the white lead (also referred to as the RA, for "Right Arm" lead) should be placed somewhere on the patient's right upper limb, preferably on the dorsal surface of the patient's right hand or wrist. The black lead (also referred to as the LA, for "Left Arm" lead) should mirror the white lead placement and be placed on the dorsal surface of the patient's left hand or wrist. The red lead (also referred to as the LL, for "Left

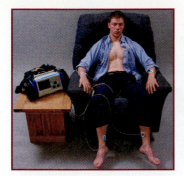

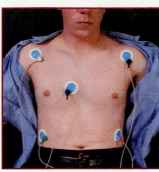

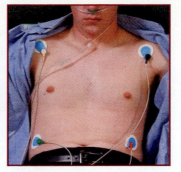

Figure 27.1   **Figure 27.2**   **Figure 27.3**

Leg" lead) should be placed on the patient's left lower limb, or on top of the left foot or near the ankle. A phrase that is often used in the prehospital setting to help with correct lead placement is "white on the right, smoke over fire."

The cardiac monitor requires at least these three electrodes to be in place in order to generate a rhythm on the oscilloscope. Depending on the lead selected (I, II, or III), these electrodes will serve as a positive electrode, negative electrode, and a ground. In a standard 4-lead application, the green lead (also referred to as the RL, for "Right Leg") is placed on the patient's right lower limb, on top of the right foot or ankle, and serves as a ground (Figure 27.1). Collectively, these leads are termed the "**limb leads.**"

Lead II is most often used when monitoring a patient's cardiac rhythm, as it allows for large, readily identifiable morphology of the P wave, QRS complex, and T wave. Modified chest lead 1 (**MCL$_1$**) is commonly used to monitor patients with atrial disturbances, as it affords a better view of electrical conduction within the atria. In MCL$_1$ the lower left (black) lead is placed in the 4th intercostal space just to the right of the sternum, and the cardiac monitor lead select is then set to Lead III (Figure 27.2).

In the prehospital environment, it is common practice for the limb leads to be placed on the anterior chest rather than the distal limbs (Figure 27.3). This placement of the electrodes causes less **artifact,** created when the patient moves his limbs or is subjected to a bumpy transport. Chest placement of the limb leads is acceptable for monitoring the cardiac rhythm in 3 leads, but a 12-lead ECG requires lead placement on the limbs to ensure accuracy.

When placing the leads and electrodes, make sure that you do not put them directly over a boney prominance and that the skin is dry, clean, and free of hair. In order to ensure good monitoring, make sure that the conducting gel is still moist when applying the patches.

Once all leads are properly placed on the patient, turn on your monitor, and confirm that you have good lead placement by switching through the different lead selections available on your monitor.

▶ EQUIPMENT

You will need the following equipment:

▶ Gloves
▶ Goggles
▶ Electrodes
▶ ECG monitor
▶ ECG leads or cables

▶ Monitor recording paper
▶ Razor or shaver (optional)
▶ Tincture of benzoin (optional)

ASSESSMENT

Place the patient in a comfortable position and perform an initial assessment, assuring that the patient has a patent airway, is breathing adequately, and has adequate circulation. Vital signs should be obtained, a focused or detailed assessment should be performed, and any life-threatening signs or symptoms should be treated immediately as they are found. Any signs, symptoms, or complaints that would suggest a possible life-threatening condition would necessitate the need for application of the cardiac monitor. In addition, some systems require cardiac monitoring, cardiac rhythm evaluation, and recording of the cardiac rhythm for patients who will be released to a BLS crew or are signing a refusal of care form.

The patient and environment should be checked for anything that could interfere with the electrical reading of the cardiac monitor such as radios and electrical appliances. The chest area of the patient should be evaluated for dirt, hair, or sweat and these conditions corrected to ensure a proper tracing. Assess the patient's pulse once the cardiac monitor is placed to make sure there is a correlation between the monitor and the pulse. The patient should be continuously reassessed.

PROCEDURE: Application of Cardiac Monitor

1. Take infection control precautions.

   Rationale: A critical patient may have the potential to vomit. Gloves and goggles are essential for preventing exposure to infectious diseases when working around critical patients, and are a must during cardiac monitoring.

2. Identify proper landmarks for lead placement. A 4-lead ECG utilizes right arm, left arm, right leg, and left leg locations for attachment of the ECG leads.

   Rationale: This lead configuration gives three possible views of the heart's electrical activity and allows for constant monitoring of the patient's cardiac rhythm.

3. Prepare the skin for lead placement. Ensure that the skin is dry, clean, and free of hair (Figure 27.4).

   Rationale: The skin should be clean and bare in the areas where leads will be placed so that the electrodes can get full contact with the skin and provide a better tracing.

4. Attach the electrodes to the leads (Figure 27.5).

   Rationale: Preparing the electrodes in advance prevents excess pressure or possible pinching of the patient's skin.

GERIATRIC NOTE:

Since geriatric patient's are more likely to suffer from illnesses that cause light tremors or shaking of the extremities, it is especially important to place the electrodes on the anterior chest and abdominal wall rather than on the distal extremities.

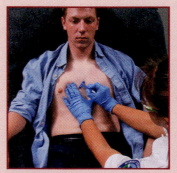

Figure 27.4

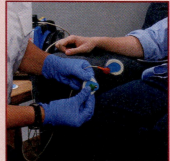

Figure 27.5

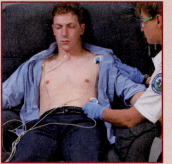
5. Place the electrodes and leads onto the prepared sites ensuring full contact with the patient's skin. Place the white lead on the right arm, the black lead on the left arm, the green lead on the right leg, and the red lead on the left leg (Figure 27.6).

   Rationale: Poor contact with the patient's skin can cause irregular tracings that can be misinterpreted as a rhythm or prevent being able to read the tracing at all.

6. Turn the power on to the cardiac monitor and adjust to Lead II if necessary (Figure 27.7).

   Rationale: Lead II is the most common lead for reading and ECG tracing, and is the lead from which cardiac treatment algorithm decisions are made. Most machines come up automatically in Lead II, but others have to manually be turned to Lead II.

7. Check the rhythm in a second lead if needed.

   Rationale: Some systems require confirmation of the ECG tracing in a second lead, either Lead I, Lead III, or MCL$_1$.

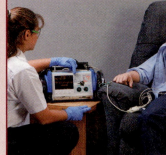

Figure 27.6

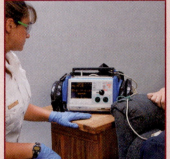

Figure 27.7

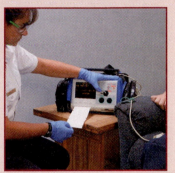

Figure 27.8

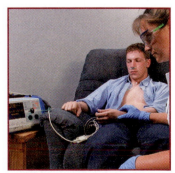

Figure 27.9

8. Interpret the ECG and discuss your findings with the patient as appropriate (Figure 27.8).

   Rationale: Rhythm interpretation helps to identify possible life-threatening patient conditions.

9. Document and record the ECG tracing by printing a strip that lasts at least 6 seconds (Figure 27.9). Attach any paper tracings that you may have to your patient care report.

   Rationale: The receiving hospital may need to confirm the initial rhythm in which the patient was found.

ONGOING ASSESSMENT

A patient who requires cardiac monitoring is either serious or unstable and should be reassessed every 5 minutes until his condition stabilizes, at which time reassessment every 15 minutes may be sufficient. Glancing at the cardiac monitor, however, is not acceptable for reassessment. A full set of vitals, including pulse, respirations, and blood pressure, in addition to cardiac rhythm interpretation, should be measured (Figure 27.10).

Resist the temptation to treat every observable rhythm. Frequently, patients will have a few unusual heart beats that require no treatment at all. If an abnormal rhythm does present on the monitor, confirm the need for treatment with other physical signs

Figure 27.10

such as changes in heart rate, respirations, blood pressure, skin color, or **diaphoresis.** Additionally, patients experiencing unusual rhythms will often complain of nausea, dizziness, or chest pain or discomfort. Act swiftly with proper treatment when needed, but only if the total patient picture warrants it.

▶PROBLEM SOLVING

▶ Proper electrode contact will be difficult in patients with much body hair. Consider shaving or clipping the hair in just that area to assist with good pad contact.

▶ Electrodes will often not adhere properly to a very diaphoretic patient. Most manufacturers make special electrodes to use on diaphoretic patients. In addition, tincture of benzoin can be used to make the electrode contact area sticky, assisting with good pad contact without interfering with the ECG tracing.

▶ Placing the leads onto the electrode pads is best done before applying the pad to the patient. To apply the lead to the pad, simply snap the button into place on the lead, and then peel off the backing to the pad and stick it on the patient in the correct location. If you place the pad and then try and attach the electrode it can be uncomfortable for the patient. You will usually have to apply a lot of downward pressure, or even pinch the skin to get the button to snap in place.

▶ Even though the leads are called "limb leads," the electrodes are commonly placed on the anterior chest. This configuration still allows for three views of the heart's electrical activity, but minimizes artifact from patient movement of the extremities. However, chest placement of the limb leads is not acceptable for 12-lead ECGs.

▶ Do not rely on the cardiac monitor to determine a patient's perfusion status. The numerical heart rate reading on the machine is measuring electrical activity only, not how many of those beats actually produce a mechanical contraction of the heart. Only mechanical contractions actually produce cardiac output and support vital body functions. Be sure to manually measure the rate, rhythm, and strength of the pulse at an arterial pulse point.

▶CASE STUDY

You arrive on scene to find a person lying prone on the floor next to his bed. The room smells of urine, and the television is turned on and quite loud. After the television is turned off, you and your paramedic partner rule out the need for c-spine and roll the patient over. As you open your airway bag, your partner checks to see that the patient is breathing and if there is a palpable pulse. He confirms that the patient is breathing 8 times per minute; has a very fast, regular pulse; and is unresponsive.

As you prepare for oxygen administration, your partner attaches electrodes to the lead cables of your monitor, and then places the leads on the patient's wrists and ankles. You turn on the monitor and see that the patient is in ventricular tachycardia. You and your partner both reconfirm that the patient has a pulse prior to reaching for the paddles and begin treatment of your unresponsive patient in ventricular tachycardia. ■

Manual Defibrillation

OBJECTIVES

The student will be able to do the following:

▶ List the indications for performing manual defibrillation
(pp. 183–184).

▶ Describe the importance of properly performing manual defibrillation
(pp. 183–184).

▶ List the steps involved in performing manual defibrillation properly
(pp. 185–187).

▶ Demonstrate the ability to perform manual defibrillation
(pp. 185–187).

INTRODUCTION

Manual defibrillation is a skill that enables you to deliver a massive amount of electricity across a patient's myocardium in an effort to stop chaotic, lethal rhythms and restore an organized, **perfusing cardiac rhythm.** Candidates for defibrillation will be those pulseless and apneic patients who present in **ventricular fibrillation (VF)** and pulseless **ventricular tachycardia (VT).** Defibrillation allows you to deliver an **unsynchronized** countershock over a time period of a few milliseconds, resulting in global depolarization of the myocardium. In effect, the defibrillation stuns the heart, producing a brief period of asystole, hopefully allowing the regular pacemaking cells of the heart in the sinoatrial node, to recover and take over control of contractile activity.

Safety is a must when employing manual defibrillation. As a trained individual you will be administering a good deal of energy to the patient. If you or anyone else is touching the patient, serious injury can occur. Once the need for defibrillation is recognized, prompt administration of an unsynchronized shock is necessary.

Defibrillation can be administered in one of two ways. One method is "hands-on" defibrillation. With this method, the **paddles** are readied and placed on the patient. While applying downward pressure on them, the patient is defibrillated. The second method, often referred to as "hands-free defibrillation." This is accomplished by using **multifunctional electrode pads,** or **MFEs,** which are very similar to AED pads. The MFEs are placed in positions that are predetermined by the manufacturer, and left in place while you take your hands off the patient and safely defibrillate by pressing buttons on the cardiac monitor. "Hands-off defibrillation" is arguably a much safer, faster, efficient, and effective method of defibrillation.

If using the paddles, several things must be accomplished prior to defibrillation. First, you must place an approved conductive medium on the paddles and make sure that the entire paddle surface is covered evenly. If using conductive jelly, it is important to ensure that gel does not smear on the skin between the paddles, or current may flow between them rather than through the chest wall and across the myocardium. If gel is not applied, you will burn the patient's skin. Second, you must find the locations for proper paddle placement. Most paddles will read Sternum or Apex. The sternum paddle should be placed near the right sternal border, near the 2nd or 3rd **intercostal space**, below the clavicle. The apex paddle should be placed near the 4th or 5th intercostal space, with the center of the paddle between the anterior and **midaxillary lines.** Do not place the paddles over large bones, any implanted defibrillator or pacemaker device or medication patches, or over the abdomen.

Next, apply approximately 25 pounds of downward pressure, making sure the paddles make good surface contact and don't slide off the patient. This is approximately the same amount of pressure you would use to provide chest compressions during CPR. Then, with the paddles in place, charge them up to the appropriate **joule** setting, look around you 360° to ensure that no one is touching the patient, look at the monitor to ensure that your patient is still in a **shockable cardiac rhythm,** yell out "I'm clear, you're clear, we're all clear" while looking up and down the patient one last time to ensure that no one is in contact, then depress the defibrillation button(s). If your monitor does not automatically record the pre- and post-shock rhythm for you, remember to press the record button on the monitor prior to and immediately after delivering the shock; this allows a printout of the intervention and patient's response, if any, to be documented.

If your monitor does not have paddles, then you will be using the MFEs. Manual defibrillation with MFEs is a very similar process, but with fewer steps. You must confirm the need for defibrillation, then dry, clean, or shave the patient's skin in the appropriate locations to ensure an adequate pad contact area. Placement of MFEs is the same as for defibrillation paddles. The package, or the MFEs themselves, will often have a diagram illustrating the locations for pad placement, should you forget. After placing the MFE pad, ensure that there is good contact between the pad and skin by smoothing out any bubbles and removing any air that is trapped between the two. Any air left between the pad and skin will undergo rapid heating and expansion during defibrillation, resulting in a burn and possible explosive detachment of the MFE pad. Do your 360° check around the patient, charge the defibrillator to the appropriate joule selection, confirm that the lethal rhythm is still present on the monitor, loudly state "I'm clear, you're clear, we're all clear" and visually ensure that this is so, then press shock and wait until the energy is released.

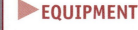

▶EQUIPMENT

You will need the following equipment (Figure 28.1):

▶ Gloves

▶ Goggles

▶ Cardiac monitor with defibrillation capability

▶ Defibrillation paddles or MFE pads

▶ Conductive gel, if paddles are to be used

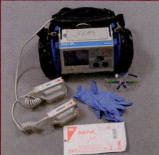

Figure 28.1

Use appropriate body substance isolation precautions. The cardiac monitor defibrillator should be checked each shift to make sure it is charged and is properly functioning. The patient should be placed in the supine position, if possible, and unresponsiveness, pulselessness, and apnea should be confirmed. In addition, the patient must be placed on the cardiac monitor or a quick look should be performed with paddles. The presence of VF or pulseless VT must be confirmed prior to defibrillation. The patient's chest should be bare and free of any liquid or substance that may act as an electrical conductor. The environment should be conducive for electrical shock, and bystander safety should be ensured. The cardiac monitor and patient should be reassessed for pulse and/or rhythm changes after each defibrillation.

PROCEDURE: Manual Defibrillation

1. Take infection control precautions.

   Rationale: A patient in sudden cardiac arrest who warrants defibrillation will commonly vomit, potentially spraying infectious airway particulates into the face of the rescuer.

2. With CPR stopped, assess for the absence of a carotid pulse and confirm that the patient is unresponsive and apneic (Figure 28.2). You should never delay CPR for more than 10 seconds to check for a pulse.

   Rationale: Defibrillation is only indicated for a patient who is pulseless and apneic.

3. Ensure that CPR is provided while you are preparing your equipment (Figure 28.3).

   Rationale: It will take some time to prepare your defibrillation equipment, and early, continuous CPR has been proven to increase the likelihood of successful defibrillation.

4. Apply conductive medium to the paddles or place defibrillation pads on the chest (Figure 28.4).

   Rationale: The conductive medium prevents burns to the patient's skin from the electricity used during defibrillation.

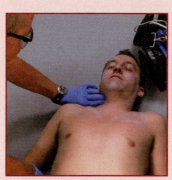

Figure 28.2

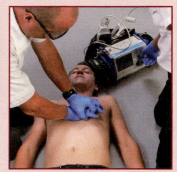

Figure 28.3

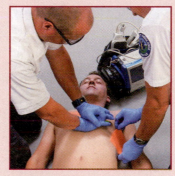

Figure 28.4

Figure 28.5

 PEDIATRIC NOTE:

All machines have either pediatric paddles or peds patches, both of which have a smaller surface area for defibrillation. For infants less than 1 year, an adult size paddle would cover too much of the chest, causing the electricity to be delivered to areas of the body other than the heart.

5. Turn the machine to "paddle" mode or turn power "on" to the paddles (Figure 28.5).

   Rationale: Since the cardiac rhythm is now being viewed by the paddles, to leave the machine in "Lead II" or other mode would prohibit reading of the rhythm when the paddles are on the chest.

continued...

GERIATRIC NOTE:

Remember that the connective tissue of the geriatric patient is more stiff and brittle, and it is not uncommon to separate the ribs from the sternum during CPR. Rib fractures generally will not interfere with your ability to defibrillate the patient.

6. Place paddles or pads in the proper position on the patient's chest using the manufacturer's suggested landmarks or the standard landmarks for the sternal pad or paddle (right sternal border at the 2nd to 3rd intercostal space inferior to the clavicle) and the apex pad or paddle (between the left anterior and midaxillary lines at the 4th to 5th intercostal space) (Figure 28.6).

   Rationale: Using proper placement of the paddles or pads ensures that the maximum amount of electricity is delivered to the fibrillating heart.

7. With CPR stopped, ensure that the cardiac monitor is displaying a shockable rhythm. Do not take longer than 10 seconds to do so (Figure 28.7).

Rationale: Only ventricular fibrillation, pulseless ventricular tachycardia, and pulseless **Torsades de Pointes** require defibrillation.

8. Select the appropriate energy level (Figure 28.8) and charge the defibrillator (Figure 28.9).

   Rationale: Whether using **monophasic** or **biphasic** defibrillators, there exists a prescribed sequence of energy levels. Choosing the proper energy level allows the most therapeutic amount of energy to be delivered to the heart without using excessive, damaging amounts of energy.

PEDIATRIC NOTE:

Pediatric patients have a much lower energy setting used for defibrillation when using both monophasic and biphasic monitors. The energy setting is based on size or weight, and therefore a Broselow® tape or other length-based resuscitation tape may be useful during the pediatric full arrest.

9. Reconfirm that the rhythm remains a shockable rhythm (Figure 28.10).

   Rationale: Defibrillating a perfusing rhythm could be lethal to the patient.

10. Order bystanders and team members to stand clear and make a 360° inspection of the patient area to ensure no persons, including you, are touching the patient. State loudly "I'm clear, you're clear, we're all clear" while confirming visually that this is true (Figure 28.11).

    Rationale: It is the responsibility of the provider performing the defibrillation to ensure that no one is in contact with the patient during the defibrillation.

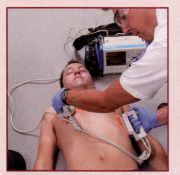

Figure 28.6

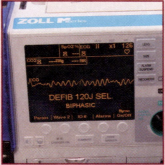

Figure 28.7

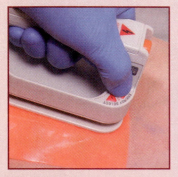

Figure 28.8

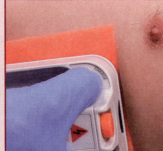

Figure 28.9

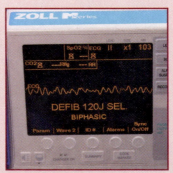

Figure 28.10

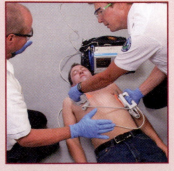

Figure 28.11

11. Press both discharge buttons simultaneously (if using paddles) or press the "shock" button if using MFEs until the unit discharges (Figure 28.12).

    Rationale: The machine will not discharge if only one of the "shock" buttons is depressed.

12. Identify post-defibrillation rhythm, and check for return of pulses if anything other than VF/VT is identified (Figure 28.13).

    Rationale: If the rhythm remains shockable, further shocks may be provided. If the defibrillation was successful in converting the rhythm, determination of the presence or lack of a pulse must be made to determine the course of care.

13. Repeat steps 7–13 as indicated by protocol if a shockable rhythm persists.

    Rationale: In some protocols, three stacked shocks are administered before interventions such as ventilation, CPR, or medication administration, while other systems use a single shock before other interventions.

14. If VF persists, following a single shock of monphasic or biphasic energy, begin CPR 30

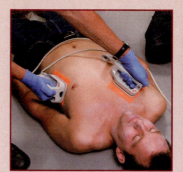 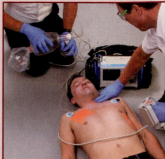

Figure 28.12   **Figure 28.13**

compressions: 2 breaths for approximately five cycles or 2 minutes.

Rationale: Newest treatment guidelines suggest a single shock before initiating other therapies is most effective.

15. Document all defibrillation attempts, including information in regards to energy levels and any rhythm changes. Attach any paper tracings that you may have to your patient care report. Include any clinical changes in the patient.

ONGOING ASSESSMENT

Reassessment of the patient who requires defibrillation requires constant vigilance to determine if he remains in cardiac arrest. The patient management priorities are numerous and include airway management, oxygenation and ventilation, suctioning of the airway, CPR, IV initiation, and medication administration. It is easy to get involved with one of the other patient management priorities and lose track of the need to reassess very simple tasks such as evaluation of pulses and respiration as indicators of return of spontaneous circulation.

Reassessment for the presence of pulses, respirations, and the cardiac rhythm displayed on the monitor should be conducted before and after every intervention such as defibrillation and medication administration. Each treatment given during cardiac arrest management is invasive, and can either be life-saving or lethal depending upon execution at just the right moment. Should an intervention appear to be successful and result in a return of spontaneous circulation, perform a full patient assessment including airway patency, breathing effort, pulses, rhythm, pulse oximetry, level of consciousness, and blood pressure.

▶PROBLEM SOLVING

▶ It is recommended that at least 25 pounds of downward pressure be applied to each of the paddles to minimize impedance during the delivery of defibrillation. This is a significant amount of pressure, and is most difficult on the apex paddle since the pressure is somewhat downward and inward.

► While MFEs can be placed in the anterior-posterior position, this is not recommended for defibrillation patches since it is likely that CPR will be in progress and the patch may interfere with hand placement during CPR. In this configuration, one MFE is placed anteriorly, to the left of the sternum directly over the heart, and the other is placed posteriorly directly behind the heart in the infrascapular region.

► The common energy shock sequence for monophasic defibrillation is 200 joules, 300 joules, 360 joules. A common energy shock sequence for biphasic defibrillation is between 120–200 joules depending on the specific manufacturer.

►CASE STUDY

It's 1:30 am, and you and your partner are in your ambulance returning to your station after a call when you are dispatched to a convalescent home for an unconscious person. A couple of minutes later, the dispatcher reports that the patient is in full arrest and that CPR is in progress. When you arrive on scene, you walk into a crowded room and see that the patient is lying supine in bed with CPR being performed by a staff member.

You clear the room of all but a few staff members who have the skills to assist, reconfirm there is no palpable pulse, and with your partner place the patient down on the ground in order to provide more effective CPR. You ask the staff member to resume CPR while your partner initiates a BLS airway and you get the defibrillator ready. You turn on the power and set the monitor to paddles, remove the paddles from the holding tray, place a quarter-size dab of gel on the conductive surface, and rub them together to ensure an even layer of gel on the surface. You tell your partner to stop CPR, and in a loud, firm voice ask everyone to get back.

You place the paddles in their proper anatomical locations, look at the monitor, and note VF. You loudly state "all clear," charge up the paddles on the patient to 200 joules, reconfirm VF on the monitor, loudly state "I'm clear, you're clear, we're all clear" while confirming visually, and then press the shock buttons and feel the paddles discharge. You immediately begin CPR, following the single shock, a complete 5 cycles of 30 compressions: 2 breaths. You look back at the monitor and note a sinus tachycardia at a rate of 124. While ventilations are continued, you feel for a carotid pulse and smile when you feel the weak, thready beat of your patient's heart. ■

CHAPTER 29

Cardioversion

KEY TERMS

Apical pulse

Atrial fibrillation

Biphasic

Brachial pulse

Cardioversion

Defibrillation

Ectopic foci

Monophasic

Paroxysmal

R wave

Supraventricular
tachycardia

Symptomatic

Synchronization

Unstable

Ventricular tachycardia

OBJECTIVES

The student will be able to do the following:

▶ List the indications for performing synchronized cardioversion (pp. 189–191).

▶ Discuss the importance of properly performing synchronized cardioversion (pp. 189–191).

▶ List and describe the proper technique of performing synchronized cardioversion (pp. 192–194).

▶ Demonstrate the ability to perform synchronized cardioversion (pp. 192–194).

INTRODUCTION

Synchronized cardioversion is the recommended treatment for a patient presenting with a hemodynamically unstable condition secondary to a tachycardic heart rhythm (except sinus tachycardia). The patient usually presents with a heart rate over 150 beats per minute with serious signs and symptoms indicating a decrease in cardiac output caused by the tachycardia. It left untreated, a patient's hemodynamic condition can deteriorate rapidly. Signs and symptoms of decreased cardiac output include hypotension, dizziness, chest pain, shortness of breath, pulmonary edema, pale, cold or diaphoretic skin, syncope, and altered level of consciousness. Depending on the severity of symptoms, a brief trial of medications may be attempted to convert the patient's heart rhythm, before the synchronized cardioversion.

Synchronized **cardioversion** is the introduction of an electrical shock across the myocardium at a specific time in the heart's conduction cycle in order to avoid the relative refractory period. It interrupts an **ectopic foci** and allows the sinus node to regain control of electrical impulse initiation. When it is effective, the heart returns to a normal rate and rhythm. Drug therapy should be attempted first, as medications are less invasive than cardioversion. Emergent cardioversion is usually reserved for the truly unstable patients or those in which drug therapy has failed. Synchronized cardioversion is only performed on patients who have a pulse; lack of a palpable pulse excludes a patient from the procedure, and the paramedic should then determine if the patient is a candidate for **defibrillation.**

When the monitor is turned to the **synchronization,** or "sync" mode, the monitor looks to capture (or mark) the top of the "R" portion of the QRS wave. This allows the shock to be delivered precisely on the peak of the **R wave,** and avoid delivery of the shock during the relative refractory period. Introducing an electrical shock during the relative refractory period (corresponding with the T wave on an ECG) can result in ventricular fibrillation, from the same mechanism that R-on-T phenomenon can result in ventricular fibrillation. Rhythms treated with synchronized cardioversion include **atrial fibrillation** and atrial flutter with rapid ventricular response, **supraventricular tachycardia,** and **ventricular tachycardia** with a pulse.

Receiving electrical intervention is painful, so if the patient is conscious and the vital signs permit you should consider administering procedural sedation per your local protocols. Procedural sedation involves pre-medicating your patient with analgesics and/or sedative hypnotic agents help your patient tolerate the procedure. Prior to any procedure, ensure your patient is appropriately monitored and all equipment is assembled and in working order. Place the patient on oxygen therapy, insert an IV line and place the patient on a cardiac and O_2 saturation monitor. Assemble your airway equipment including a BVM device, suction, and intubation equipment in case the patient cardiac arrests.

In addition, taking the time to explain the procedure to the patient may help relieve some of the fear and stress that accompanies the procedure. In cases of tachydysrhythmias resulting in severe hemodynamic compromise, synchronized cardioversion may need to take place immediately without the benefit of premedication and explanation; in such cases, it is not uncommon for the patient to have a decreased level of consciousness or be completely unconscious, making communication impossible anyway.

The energy selection, or joules settings, begins lower than that of defibrillation. There are specific AHA recommendations for joule settings and they are used in the table below for reference. The settings may be different if a **biphasic** defibrillator is used as it often requires less energy than a **monophasic** defbrillator. Check your local protocols and manufacturer settings for proper joule settings.

Identified Rhythm	Recommended Monophasic Joules*
Atrial Fibrillation	100J, 200J, 300J, 360J
Atrial Flutter	50J, 100J, 200J, 300J, 360J
Supraventricular Tachcardia (SVT)	50J, 100J, 200J, 300J, 360J
	SVT often responds to lower energy levels
Polymorphic Ventricular Tachycardia (VT)	200J, 300J, 360J
	Treat as if this were VF with high energy levels
Stable Ventricular Tachycardia (VT)	100J, 200J, 300J, 360J

*Consult the individual manufacturer recommendations for biphasic joules equivalents. The biphasic joule equivalent is often lower and varies dependent upon the type of biphasic waveform.

One potentially deadly mistake made with synchronized cardioversion is failure to press the sync button on the monitor prior to cardioversion. If the sync button is not pressed, then the monitor will deliver an unsynchronized shock equivalent to a defibrillation that may fall during the relative refractory period and cause the onset of ventricular fibrillation. You must remember to press the sync button before each synchronized cardioversion, as most defibrillators will default back to the defibrillation, or unsynchronized, mode once a synchronized shock has been delivered. In effect, you would then be defibrillating your patient.

As the computer will not deliver the electricity until an R wave has been positively identified, it may take several seconds for the monitor to release the energy. You may have to hold down the discharge buttons longer than you would with unsynchronized shocks (defibrillation). The computer is simply looking for the best R wave to deliver the electricity, assuring that the delivery does not occur during the relative refractory period.

After synchronized cardioversion, check the monitor, patient's responsiveness and pulse. If the rhythm continues to be rapid, and the patient is still **symptomatic,** or **unstable,** then synchronized cardioversion must be performed again. Turn on the sync mode on the monitor, confirm that the monitor is capturing the peak of the R waves (usually indicated by a dot or arrow atop each R-wave on the screen) charge up the monitor to the required joule setting, then press and hold the shock buttons until the cardioversion is delivered.

▶ EQUIPMENT

You will need the following equipment:

- ▶ Gloves
- ▶ Goggles
- ▶ Cardiac monitor with cardioversion capabilities
- ▶ ECG electrodes
- ▶ ECG lead cables
- ▶ Defibrillation/cardioversion pads or paddles
- ▶ IV line and fluids
- ▶ O_2 saturation monitor
- ▶ O_2 nasal cannula or mask
- ▶ BVM
- ▶ Intubation equipment
- ▶ Sedative medication (optional)

ASSESSMENT

Use appropriate body substance isolation precautions. The cardiac monitor/ defibrillator should be checked each shift to make sure it is charged and is functioning properly.

Place the patient in the supine position, and perform an initial assessment to ensure that the patient has a patent airway, is breathing adequately, and has adequate circulation. Place the patient on continuous cardiac monitoring and an O_2 saturation monitor. Due to the hemodynamic instability that often accompanies tachycardic dysrhythmias, there is a high likelihood that aggressive airway maintenance and ventilation with supplemental oxygen will be required. Assess the patient's respiratory function by listening to breath sounds and observing the rate, depth, and effort of breathing. Place the patient on high-flow oxygen keeping the O_2 saturation above 95 percent. Assess the patient's hemodynamic status by monitoring the patient's blood pressure, pulse rate and quality, and cardiac rhythm. Place a large bore IV in anticipation of fluid resuscitation or medications. Observe the skin for temperature, diaphoresis and color as pale or cyanotic. Prepare for cardioversion if the assessment findings confirm the patient is hemodynamically unstable.

In addition, complaints such as chest pain, dizziness, and syncope may influence the decision to perform cardioversion. Obtain a complete set of vital signs. In addition a detailed assessment, determination of the dysrhythmia should be performed to confirm that cardioversion is appropriate. Prior to cardioversion, you should ensure that the environment is safe for cardioversion. For example, no water should be touching the patient, and, further, no rescuers should be in contact with the patient.

The patient should be reassessed immediately after each cardioversion and continuously monitored.

PROCEDURE: Cardioversion

1. Take infection control precautions.

   Rationale: It is not uncommon for unstable patients who need cardioversion to vomit, spraying potentially infectious material into the mucous membranes of the rescuer.

2. Apply the monitor leads to the patient. The patient must be continuously monitored in Lead I, II or III, and not "paddles" for this procedure.

   Rationale: Continuous cardiac monitoring in one of the standard three leads is necessary for this procedure.

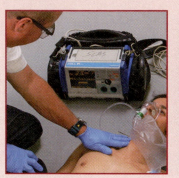
Figure 29.1

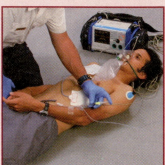
Figure 29.2

3. Confirm the dysrhythmia, and assess for the presence of a carotid pulse (Figure 29.1).

   Rationale: Only patients who have pulses are candidates for cardioversion.

PEDIATRIC NOTE:

Many pediatric patients have fleshy necks, making a carotid pulse more difficult to assess. Determination of a **brachial pulse** is indicated for infants, while an **apical pulse** can also be used to confirm the presence of a pulse. Other signs of poor perfusion should be assessed such as skin color, temperature, and capillary refill time.

4. Apply O₂ by cannula or face mask and monitor the patient's oxygen saturation. Assemble advanced airway equipment in the event more aggressive airway management is needed.

   Rationale: Respiratory compromise and arrest may accompany hemodynamic instability or a failed cardioversion attempt.

5. Establish an IV or saline lock for medication or fluid administration.

   Rationale: IV fluid boluses may be required for the hemodynamically unstable patient in order to maintain blood pressure. Antidysrythmic medications may be attempted before cardioversion to chemically convert the patient.

6. Explain the procedure to the patient, and sedate the patient as needed (Figure 29.2).

   Rationale: Cardioversion can be a frightening and painful experience for the patient. If the patient is alert and oriented, consider sedation with analgesics, sedatives, or hypnotics.

PEDIATRIC NOTE:

It is well documented in the medical literature that children are not assessed properly for pain, and are treated less often and less aggressively for pain management. The electrical current from a cardioversion is going to hurt, and if the child is alert at all, sedation should be used.

7. Turn on the defibrillation/cardioversion function of the cardiac monitor (Figure 29.3).

   Rationale: The power will need to be turned on to discharge the electricity and perform the cardioversion.

8. Apply conductive medium to paddles or place defibrillation/cardioversion pads on the bare chest (Figure 29.4).

   Rationale: The conductive medium prevents burns to the patient's skin from the electricity used during cardioversion.

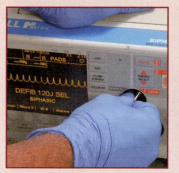

Figure 29.3

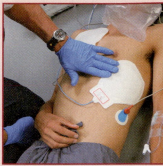

Figure 29.4

> ### GERIATRIC NOTE:
>
> Because declining body systems cause geriatric patients to have poor thermoregulatory mechanisms, they often tend to be dressed in more layers of clothing. If you have any suspicion that your patient may decompensate and require cardioversion or defibrillation, disrobe the patient from the waist up to prevent the clothes from hindering your access to the chest. In addition, consider applying defibrillation/cardioversion pads to the patient's chest prior to the onset of dysrhythmia, allowing for a more rapid delivery of the counter shock.

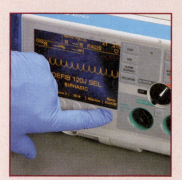

Figure 29.5

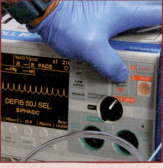

Figure 29.6

9. Press the "sync" button on the monitor and confirm the "R" wave is being sensed by the computer by observing markers on the "R" waves (Figure 29.5).

   Rationale: This assures that the energy will only be delivered on a recognized R wave, avoiding the relative refractory period and providing a true synchronized cardioversion and not a defibrillation.

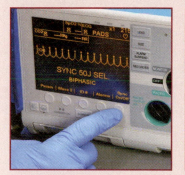

Figure 29.7

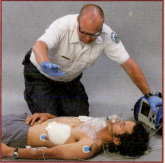

Figure 29.8

10. Ensure paddles or pads are in the proper position on the patient's chest using the manufacturer's suggested landmarks or the standard landmarks of the patient's right sternal border (around the 2nd intercostal space) and the left anterior axillary line (about the 5th intercostal space).

    Rationale: Using proper placement of the pads or paddles ensures that the maximum amount of electricity is delivered to the myocardium.

11. Select the appropriate energy level and charge the unit (Figure 29.6).

    Rationale: Whether using monophasic or biphasic monitors for cardioversion, there exists a prescribed sequence of energy levels. Choosing the proper energy level allows the most

therapeutic amount of energy to be delivered to the heart without using excessive or damaging amounts of energy.

12. Reconfirm that the rhythm requires cardioversion and that the machine is in "sync" mode by noting the markers on the "R" waves (Figure 29.7).

    Rationale: Many rhythms are **paroxysmal,** and may have corrected themselves before cardioversion could be initiated.

13. Order bystanders and team members to stand clear and make a 360° inspection of the patient area to ensure no persons, including yourself, are touching the patient (Figure 29.8).

continued...

Rationale: Any person in contact with the patient during cardioversion will also receive the electricity, which will not only be painful, but may potentially result in life-threatening dysrhythmia.

14. Press both discharge buttons simultaneously (if using paddles) or press the "shock" button if using patches until the unit discharges. Hold paddles in place until the energy is delivered.

    Rationale: Since the machine is delivering a synchronized cardioversion, it will not actually discharge the energy until an adequate R wave is identified. Moving the paddles before the energy is discharged will result in a failed cardioversion attempt.

15. Identify the post-cardioversion rhythm and check for the presence of pulses (Figure 29.9).

    Rationale: Cardioversion is used to abort a dangerous rhythm that is not allowing the heart to produce adequate cardiac output. Following cardioversion, you would expect to see a more controlled heart rate, rise in blood pressure, and improvement of symptoms reported by the patient.

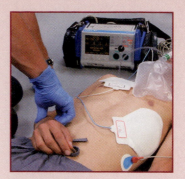

Figure 29.9

16. Repeat steps 9–15 as indicated by protocol if rhythm persists.

    Rationale: Subsequent cardioversions at higher energy settings may be needed if the rhythm is not converted.

17. Document all cardioversion attempts, including information in regards to energy levels and any rhythm changes. Attach any paper tracings that you may have to your patient care report. Include any clinical changes in the patient.

ONGOING ASSESSMENT

In the event that synchronized cardioversion was successful in converting a tachy-dysrhythmia to a more stable rhythm, it will be necessary to continue assessing your patient. Obtain a full set of vital signs immediately after the procedure to ensure that your patient has a patent airway, is breathing adequately, and has a pulse that not only corresponds with the rhythm generated on the cardiac monitor, but supports an adequate cardiac output as well. If cardioversion has resulted in successful rhythm conversion, you should expect to find a general improvement in the patient's hemodynamic state. Remember that any analgesics, sedatives, or hypnotics administered prior to cardioversion may affect the patient long after conversion, resulting in the need for airway control or assisted ventilations. Inspect the patient's chest for any burning that may have occurred during the procedure. Pain control may be required after cardioversion as well.

In cases where cardioversion is unsuccessful in converting the patient out of the tachydysrhythmia, the airway, breathing, and circulation must be reassessed continuously to prevent further compromise.

▶PROBLEM SOLVING

▶ The "sync" function is automatically turned off by the monitor after every cardioversion, requiring that you reset the function for each subsequent cardioversion. This is intended as a safety feature for the patient in case the cardioversion accidentally puts the patient into a lethal ventricular fibrillation. Since ventricular fibrillation is an irregularly irregular rhythm, if the sync button were on, the machine would never discharge the electricity, possibly resulting in an unacceptable delay of defibrillation to the patient.

▶ Stimulation of the vagus nerve may terminate the tachydysrythmia, eliminating the need for cardioversion. Some systems have the patient bear down or blow forcefully through pursed lips to try to stimulate the vagas nerve before deciding to use cardioversion.

▶ When possible, it is prudent to sedate a patient with an analgesic, sedative, hypnotic agent, or combination thereof prior to cardioversion. However, if the patient is altered, there is no need to sedate him or her first. In fact, an altered level of consciousness is a contraindication to most sedatives.

▶CASE STUDY

You are working on a paramedic engine and are dispatched to the local park for a reported man down. As you arrive on scene, you confirm that there are no hazards to you or your team, and notice an elderly man lying supine in the middle of a soccer field. As you approach the patient you note that he appears to be in his mid 50s, is very pale and diaphoretic, and does not respond when you call to him. After ruling out the need for c-spine precautions, you perform a painful stimuli, but there is still no response. The patient is breathing at a rate of 20/min and you feel that he has a very weak, rapid, and regular carotid pulse.

As your partner applies a nonrebreather oxygen mask, you hook up the monitor and note that the patient is in a supraventricular tachycardia at a rate of 240 bpm. Your partner exposes the patient's chest as you apply some conducting gel to the defibrillation paddles, press the sync button, and place the paddles on the patient's chest. You see that the computer is identifying the R wave of each QRS complex, charge up the monitor to 50 joules, and reconfirm the patient's rhythm, unresponsiveness, and presence of a pulse. After yelling "all clear" and visually ensuring that everyone is clear of the patient, you hold down the shock buttons until the energy is released. You reassess your patient and monitor. The monitor now shows a sinus tachycardia at a rate of 116 bpm that corresponds with a carotid pulse, and the patient slowly opens his eyes. ■

CHAPTER 30

External Cardiac Pacing

KEY TERMS

Asystole

Bradycardia

Capture

Heart blocks

Milliamp (mA)

Multifunctional electrode pads (MFEs)

Overdrive pacing

Pacer spike

Poor perfusion

Pulse per minute (PPM)

Pulseless electrical activity (PEA)

OBJECTIVES

The student will be able to do the following:

▶ List the indications for performing external cardiac pacing (pp. 196–197).
▶ Describe the importance of properly performing external cardiac pacing (pp. 196–197).
▶ List and describe the steps involved in the proper technique for performing external cardiac pacing (pp. 197–199).
▶ Demonstrate the ability to perform external cardiac pacing (pp. 197–199).

INTRODUCTION

External cardiac pacing is a skill that allows you to control a patient's heart rate from outside his body. Electrodes placed on the skin deliver electrical impulses from the pulse generator located within a cardiac monitor through the thoracic tissue to the heart, resulting in depolarization of the myocardium and cardiac muscle contraction. As such, the pulse generator of a pacing unit takes over pacemaking duties from the SA node. This skill must be used with a pacing capable monitor and trained individual.

External cardiac pacing is indicated when the patient complains or shows signs of **poor perfusion** due to **bradycardia.** Pacing is a Class I recommendation for hemodynamically unstable bradycardia and also AMI with the following rhythms—symptomatic sinus node dysfunction, 2nd degree type II AV block, 3rd degree AV block, new left, right, or alternating bundle branch block (BBB) or bifascicular block. The most common rhythms that are paced are symptomatic bradycardia, bradycardia that was witnessed to degenerate into **asystole,** cardiac arrest with **pulseless electrical activity (PEA)** secondary to drug overdose, electrolyte abnormalities, or acidosis, and **heart blocks.** Symptomatic means that the slow heart rate is causing the patient to experience signs and symptoms like chest pain, shortness of breath, hypotension, poor skin signs, or even an altered level of consciousness (ALOC). Any time a patient suffers from symptomatic bradycardia, consider less invasive maneuvers first while preparing to pace. If that proves unsuccessful then move directly to external cardiac pacing to correct the bradycardia. Some sources recommend that if a high degree heart block exists you should go directly to pacing and avoid administering atropine. High degree heart blocks consist of 2nd degree type II and 3rd degree heart blocks.

Precautions

As this procedure can be the source of significant, repetitive pain, the paramedic should consider the administration of analgesic, sedative, or hypnotic medication prior to initiation of pacing, if possible. If the patient is unconscious and/or significantly unstable, you may have to initiate external cardiac pacing prior to medication administration.

External cardiac pacing is contraindicated for prolonged bradyasystolic cardiac arrest. Pacing is also contraindicated for the severely hypothermic patient. The patient should be warmed first and then reassessed for pacing.

Pacing is achieved by using large conductive pads, or **multifunctional electrode pads (MFEs),** adhered to the patient's chest. They are very sticky, and expensive, so make sure before you put them on the patient's chest that you are putting them in the right locations. Before actually placing the pads, you may have to clean, dry, or even shave the chest area. The pads work best when there is as much pad-to-skin contact as possible. Any impedance can alter the performance of the pads and result in burns to the contact area.

Placement of the MFEs works best in an anterior-posterior position over the apex of the heart. Place the anterior electrode over the apex of the heart, just to the left of the sternum. The posterior electrode should be placed to the left of the thoracic spinal column between the shoulder blades. This will allow the electricity to flow directly through the heart most efficiently. If you ever forget, just look at the package or pads, as most manufacturers suggest where to place them on the patient with a convenient diagram.

When the monitor is turned to the pacing function, you will need to adjust the **pulse per minute (PPM),** or pulse rate, and the **milliamp (mA)** output. The PPM allows you to adjust to the desired heart rate, and the mA output allows for either an increase or decrease in electrical output. A good PPM to start out with is between 60 and 80 beats per minute. When dealing with the mA, make sure that you start out at low mA, and then slowly increase the output until you see capture. Don't be afraid to touch the patient, as it is not enough electricity to harm yourself or others.

The presence of a **pacer spike,** seen as a vertical line, followed by a wide, unusual-looking QRS complex, indicates **capture.** The QRS complex following the pacer spike will be abnormally wide, as the electrical impulse is not following the normal conduction pathway through the ventricles. Once you believe that you have capture on the monitor, check for a pulse and make sure that it correlates with the monitor rate.

Just because the monitor shows electrical capture does not mean that you will also have mechanical capture. If pacing does not work, then disable the pacer and move on with other drug therapies. The pacer will not show atrial capture, only ventricular capture. At this point, your patient's need for sedation, if he has not yet been medicated, will become quite evident and should be promptly addressed. Continued sedation will be required throughout the duration of the procedure.

Oxygen administration and IV access should be initiated in all patients prior to external cardiac pacing, if possible. Those patients who are significantly unstable may require pacing prior to IV access. Efforts should be made to initiate IV access as soon as possible after pacing is started.

▶ EQUIPMENT

You will need the following equipment:

- ▶ Gloves
- ▶ Goggles
- ▶ Cardiac monitor with pacing capabilities
- ▶ ECG electrodes
- ▶ Pacing patches or multifunctional electrodes

ASSESSMENT

Patients requiring external cardiac pacing, first and foremost, will present with bradycardia. Not all bradycardia, however, requires pacing; only those patients who are hemodynamically unstable as a result of their bradycardia should be paced. Indications of hemodynamic instability include altered mental status; hypotension; cool, pale, diaphoretic skin; cyanosis; delayed capillary refill; the development of pulmonary edema; and any other sign suggestive of decreased cardiac output and poor perfusion. In addition, patient complaints of chest pain, dizziness, weakness, shortness of breath, syncope, and nausea/vomiting should suggest the need for external cardiac pacing.

PROCEDURE: External Cardiac Pacing

1. Take infection control precautions.

   Rationale: It is not uncommon for patients with severe symptomatic bradycardia to feel nauseated and vomit, spraying potentially infectious material into the face and mucous membranes of the rescuer.

2. Confirm that the rhythm on the monitor and the clinical condition of the patient both indicate that use of external cardiac pacing is warranted (Figure 30.1).

   Rationale: In general, pacing is only indicated for very slow rhythms that result in poor perfusion and some patients in cardiac arrest.

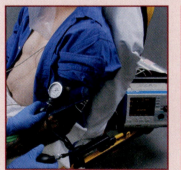

Figure 30.1   **Figure 30.2**

▶ PEDIATRIC NOTE:

Bradycardic rhythms in children are usually the result of a respiratory problem, not an underlying cardiac condition. Be sure all airway issues such as opening the airway, suctioning, oxygenation, and ventilation are accomplished before moving into any electrical therapy.

3. If the patient is conscious, explain the procedure and offer sedation prior to initiation of external cardiac pacing (Figure 30.2).

   Rationale: This procedure may be frightening and produce some discomfort. The patient, if conscious and coherent, will be more cooperative and compliant if he is aware of what to expect.

4. Apply pacing pads onto the bare chest using anterior-posterior position or following the manufacturer's recommendation (Figures 30.3 and 30.4).

   Rationale: The typical position for pacing pads is A-P; however, some multifunctional pads allow for an apex-base placement.

5. Turn the machine to "paddle" mode or turn the power "on" to the pacer (Figure 30.5).

   Rationale: Since the ECG rhythm is now being viewed by the pacing patches, the machine would be unable to display the rhythm in Lead II.

6. Set the desired heart rate on the pacer to approximately 80 beats per minute (Figure 30.6).

   Rationale: A heart rate between 60 and 80 beats per minute is considered acceptable.

7. Dial up the energy in small increments of milliamps until consistent mechanical and electrical capture is observed (Figure 30.7). Electrical capture is observed when a pacemaker spike is present on the ECG along with widening of the QRS complex and broadening of the T-wave.

   Rationale: Failure to maintain electrical or mechanical capture will result in further deterioration of the patient's condition.

8. Assess the patient for pulses that are consistent with the paced rhythm on the cardiac monitor (Figure 30.8).

   Rationale: If the pacing is indeed successful, then a mechanical contraction should be felt as a radial pulse.

9. Once electrical and mechanical capture have been achieved, add 2 mA as a safety margin.

   Rationale: Mechanical capture is indicated by a pulse that is synchronous with the paced beat.

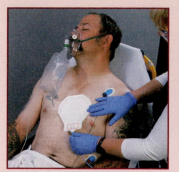
Figure 30.3

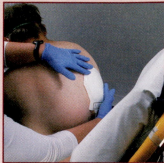
Figure 30.4

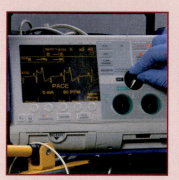
Figure 30.5

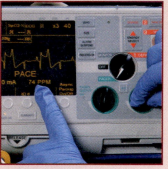
Figure 30.6

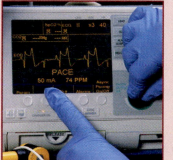

Figure 30.7

Figure 30.8

continued...

10. Reassess the patient frequently for maintenance of capture and return of an underlying perfusing rhythm (Figure 30.9).

Rationale: Successful pacing sometimes resets the heart's underlying rhythm and will result in an adequate number of perfusing beats from the patient. Contact medical control, however, if the pacer is to be discontinued.

11. Initiate CPR if capture is not observed when at the maximum energy setting and no pulse is palpated.

Rationale: Only when capture is observed will the heart be producing mechanical contractions. If capture is not observed and the patient was initially in asystole or PEA, then CPR will be required.

12. Document all information regarding the pacing attempts, including information in regards to

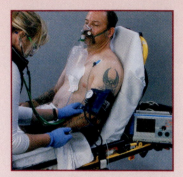

Figure 30.9

milliamps need for capture and any rhythm changes. Attach any paper tracings that you may have to your PCR. Include any clinical changes in the patient.

ONGOING ASSESSMENT

A patient who requires pacing is unstable, with serious signs and symptoms of poor perfusion. In most cases, the pacer is applied only after medication therapy has failed. Therefore, frequent reassessment for both improvements and deterioration is necessary. A proper reassessment includes measurement of vital signs including blood pressure, peripheral pulses, respirations, lung sounds, skin signs, and level of consciousness.

Many patients will initially appear much better after pacing has begun and capture is achieved. Often, as a result of improved perfusion, peripheral pulses and a blood pressure will be measurable. Skin signs will also improve, as will the level of consciousness. However, do not be fooled into thinking that the conduction problem with the heart is fixed. Do not remove the pacer! All of the improvements witnessed are a direct result of the pacer, and will quickly reverse themselves if the pacer is removed.

▶ PROBLEM SOLVING

▶ This skill addresses only the pacing of slow, nonperfusing rhythms. It is possible to conduct "**overdrive pacing**" of an unstable tachycardia with a pacer. However, this is not typically used in the prehospital setting.

▶ Since pacing is only used on an unstable patient, there is usually no need to sedate the patient prior to application of the pacer. Usually, patients who require pacing already have an altered level of consciousness. However, if the patient does complain of discomfort from the pacer, an analgesic or sedative such as morphine, diazepam, or midazolam may be considered.

▶ There is no need to "clear" bystanders or rescuers prior to the application of the pacer. The energy delivered is different than that used during cardioversion and defibrillation, and is not harmful to the rescuer. It will be possible to feel the pacer, but it is not painful. The sensation feels like a tingling sensation during CPR or other patient treatments.

▶CASE STUDY

You are working on a dual paramedic ALS ambulance and are returning from your morning drills when you receive a call for a possible unconscious person at a bus stop. You arrive on scene and ask the first-responding fire unit to block traffic and assure scene safety. You and your partner approach what looks like a transient sitting on the bench, slumped over. When you yell out to him, he does not respond. You perform a painful stimulus, and the patient swings his arm at you. As you begin to talk and assess the patient, you realize that his only complaint is that he cannot stay awake. You check his pulse and realize that it is very slow.

As you continue to assess and talk to the patient, he slumps over again. You arouse the patient again, and he questions you as to what is going on. You place the patient on your cardiac monitor and immediately note a reading of Mobitz II. You immediately tell the patient what is going on, and what you are going to do, while placing him on the gurney. The patient's blood pressure is above 100 systolic so you call the base hospital and get an order to premedicate this patient with 5 mg of versed IV push. You administer oxygen to the patient with a nonrebreather mask, establish IV access, place the MFEs in the proper A-P locations, and administer the 5 mg of versed.

Once you note that the versed is taking effect, you turn the pacer on, set the pulse per minute rate at 70, and being to turn the milliamps up in small increments. You recognize capture at around 92 mA, with a pacer spike preceding a wide QRS, and immediately feel for a pulse. You feel a radial pulse that corresponds with the monitor, and also note that every third pacer spike is not capturing. You increase the energy to 100 mA and note complete capture; any attempt to lower the energy selection results in the occasional dropped beat, so you leave it at 100 mA. The patient has a good, regular pulse; is conscious and alert; and is transported to the hospital without any other complications. ■

CHAPTER 31

Application of a 12-Lead ECG Monitor

KEY TERMS

Artifact

Augmented limb leads

Diaphoresis

Electrode

Leads

Limb leads

Precordial, or chest, leads

OBJECTIVES

The student will be able to do the following:

▶ List the indications for application of a 12-lead cardiac monitor (pp. 202–204).

▶ Describe the importance of proper application of a 12-lead cardiac monitor (pp. 202–204).

▶ Describe the proper technique involved in the application of a 12-lead cardiac monitor (pp. 205–207).

▶ Demonstrate the ability to apply a 12-lead cardiac monitor (pp. 205–207).

INTRODUCTION

Once considered an exotic piece of diagnostic equipment of no use to the paramedic, the 12-lead ECG is now commonly used in the prehospital environment, and with good reason. The 12-lead ECG allows for the early identification of developing myocardial ischemia, allowing the paramedic and medical control to make prompt and appropriate treatment and transport determinations. The initiation of fibrinolytic therapy or cardiac catheterization relies on accurate 12-lead ECG interpretation, and early identification of candidates can significantly reduce the "identification to medication" (or door-to-cath lab) time in these patients. The diagnostic accuracy of the 12-lead ECG is heavily dependant on proper lead placement.

A 12-lead ECG requires the placement of 10 **leads**: 4 **limb leads** and 6 **precordial, or chest, leads**. The limb leads, which produce Leads I, II, and III, should be placed on the limbs, at least 10 cm from the heart, and avoid any bony prominences that may interfere with electrical conduction. Specifically, the right arm lead (RA, white) and left arm lead (LA, black) should be placed between the shoulder and wrist parallel to each other, and the right leg lead (RL, green) and left leg lead (LL, red) should be placed between the hip and ankle parallel to each other.

While the limb leads can be placed over any fleshy area on the appropriate extremity, it is common to use the bicep for the upper limb leads and the thigh or calf for the lower limb leads (Figure 31.1). Limb leads placed on the wrists and ankles have a higher risk of creating **artifact,** as patient movement is exaggerated at the distal limbs compared to the proximal. While placing limb leads on the chest is acceptable for routine monitoring, a diagnostic-quality 12-lead ECG requires that the limb leads be placed on the limbs; if a 12-lead ECG is generated using limb leads placed on the patient's torso, a note should be made on the ECG stating such.

In addition to Leads I, II, and III, the limb leads are manipulated by the ECG computer to produce the augmented voltage (aV) leads: aVR (right arm), aVL (left arm), and aVF (foot). The computer performs vector manipulation of the limb leads to combine two selected limb leads, essentially producing an "**electrode**" in the center of the heart that, when combined with the remaining limb lead, gives an additional view of the heart. As there are three limb leads, three **augmented limb leads** are generated.

The precordial leads, also called vector (V) leads, comprise the last 6 leads of a 12-lead ECG and are placed across the chest in specific locations (Figure 31.2) (Table 31.1). As proper placement of the precordial leads is necessary for the generation of an accurate 12-lead ECG recording, it is absolutely necessary that the paramedic is familiar with and able to identify the exact location for each lead placement. Guessing, estimating, or "eye-balling" 12-lead ECG electrode placement is unacceptable, and will result in inaccurate ECG tracings and erroneous interpretations.

The most common method for identifying the proper electrode attachment sites utilizes a familiar landmark on the sternum, the Angle of Louis. The first rib articulates with the sternum at the Angle of Louis, allowing for identification of the 1st intercostal space immediately inferior to the 1st rib. Simply "counting down" the subsequent intercostal spaces allows for rapid identification of the 4th intercostal space, the location for Leads V_1 and V_2. After location identification and placement of these leads, V_3–V_6 can be easily placed as described in Table 31.1.

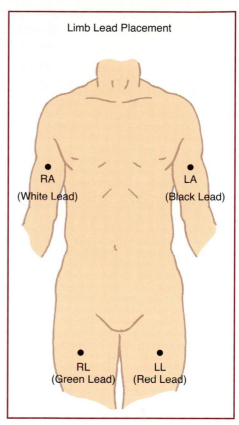

Limb Lead Placement

RA
(White Lead)

LA
(Black Lead)

RL
(Green Lead)

LL
(Red Lead)

Figure 31.1

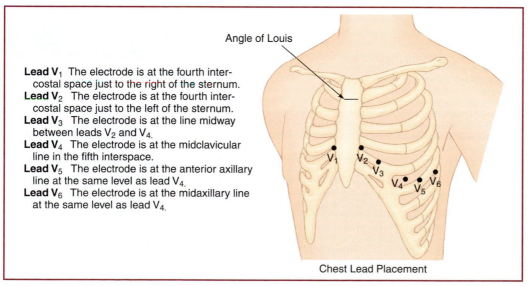

Angle of Louis

Lead V_1 The electrode is at the fourth intercostal space just to the right of the sternum.
Lead V_2 The electrode is at the fourth intercostal space just to the left of the sternum.
Lead V_3 The electrode is at the line midway between leads V_2 and V_4.
Lead V_4 The electrode is at the midclavicular line in the fifth interspace.
Lead V_5 The electrode is at the anterior axillary line at the same level as lead V_4.
Lead V_6 The electrode is at the midaxillary line at the same level as lead V_4.

V_1 V_2 V_3
V_4 V_5 V_6

Chest Lead Placement

Figure 31.2

TABLE 31.1	Chest Lead Placement
Lead	Placement
V_1	Fourth intercostal space, just to the right of the sternum
V_2	Fourth intercostal space, just to the left of the sternum
V_3	Between V_2 and V_4
V_4	Fifth intercostal space, midclavicular line
V_5	Anterior axillary line, level with V_4
V_6	Midaxillary line, level with V_4 and V_5

As with the cardiac monitor (Chapter 27), ensure that the ECG electrodes are not placed directly over a bony prominence and that the skin is dry, clean, and free of hair. In order to ensure good monitoring, make sure that the conducting gel is still moist when applying the electrodes. In addition, tincture of benzoin can be utilized to increase electrode adherence if the patient is diaphoretic.

Indications for performing a 12-lead ECG include the suspicion of myocardial ischemia and the need for rhythm interpretation as determined by a review of the patient's past medical history (PMH), chief complaint, history of present illness (HPI), clinical exam findings, diagnostic exam findings, or any combination thereof. There are no contraindications to 12-lead ECG determination. In most systems patients complaining of chest pain, shortness of breath, weakness or syncope will all have a 12-lead performed.

►EQUIPMENT

You will need the following equipment (Figure 31.3):

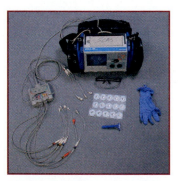

▶ Gloves

▶ Goggles

▶ Electrodes

▶ 12-lead ECG monitor

▶ 12-lead ECG leads or cables

▶ Monitor recording paper

▶ Razor or shaver (optional)

▶ Tincture of benzoin (optional)

Figure 31.3

ASSESSMENT

Place the patient in a comfortable position and perform an initial assessment, assuring that the patient has a patent airway, is breathing adequately, and has adequate circulation. Obtain vital signs, perform a focused and detailed assessment, and treat any life-threatening signs or symptoms immediately as they are found. Any findings in the patient's PMH, chief complaint, HPI, clinical exams, or diagnostic exams that would suggest a possible life-threatening cardiac condition would indicate the need for 12-lead ECG interpretation.

The patient and environment should be checked for anything that could interfere with the acquisition of the 12-lead ECG such as radios and electrical appliances. The chest and limbs of the patient should be evaluated for ease of application of cardiac electrodes, and a razor or tincture of benzoin used to prepare the skin if excessive hair or **diaphoresis** is present, respectively. Assess the patient's pulse once the cardiac monitor is placed and prior to the 12-lead ECG determination to make sure there is a correlation between the monitor and the pulse. The patient should be continuously reassessed.

PROCEDURE: Application of 12-Lead ECG Monitor

1. Take infection control precautions.
   Rationale: Gloves and goggles are essential for preventing exposure to infectious diseases when working around critical patients, and are required during 12-lead ECG electrode placement.

2. Prepare the skin for limb and precordial lead placement. Ensure that the skin is dry, clean, and free of hair (Figure 31.4).
   Rationale: The skin should be clean and bare in the areas where leads will be placed so that the electrodes can get full contact with the skin and provide a better tracing.

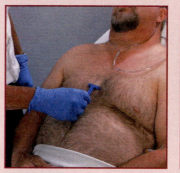
Figure 31.4

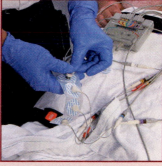
Figure 31.5

> **PEDIATRIC NOTE:**
> ECG tracings will be more accurate if properly sized leads are used. Both neonate and pediatric electrodes exist and should be used on smaller patients.

3. Attach the electrodes to the leads (Figure 31.5).
   Rationale: Preparing the electrodes in advance avoids the need to press on the patient with excessive pressure.

4. Identify proper locations for limb lead placement.
   Rationale: This lead configuration provides the three limb leads and three augmented limb lead views of the heart's electrical activity and also allows for constant monitoring of the patient's cardiac rhythm in Lead II.

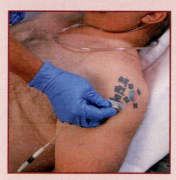
Figure 31.6

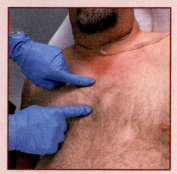
Figure 31.7

5. Place the limb leads onto the prepared sites ensuring full contact with the patient's skin and avoiding bony prominences. Place one lead on the right arm, another on the left arm (Figure 31.6), another lead on the right leg, and the last lead on the left leg.
   Rationale: Improperly placed or poorly adhered electrodes can affect the quality and accuracy of the 12-lead ECG tracing.

6. Prepare for precordial lead placement by identifying the 4th intercostal space, using the Angle of Louis on the sternum to identify the 1st rib and intercostal space (Figure 31.7).
   Rationale: The use of known landmarks to identify the proper lead attachment sites is highly recommended to ensure an accurate 12-lead ECG tracing.

> **GERIATRIC NOTE:**
> Since geriatric patients are more likely to suffer from illnesses that cause light tremors or shaking of the extremities, it may be necessary to place the electrodes on the bicep rather than the wrist to reduce artifact.

continued...

PROCEDURE: Application of 12-Lead ECG Monitor (continued)

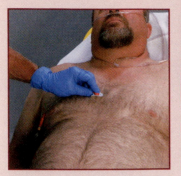

Figure 31.8

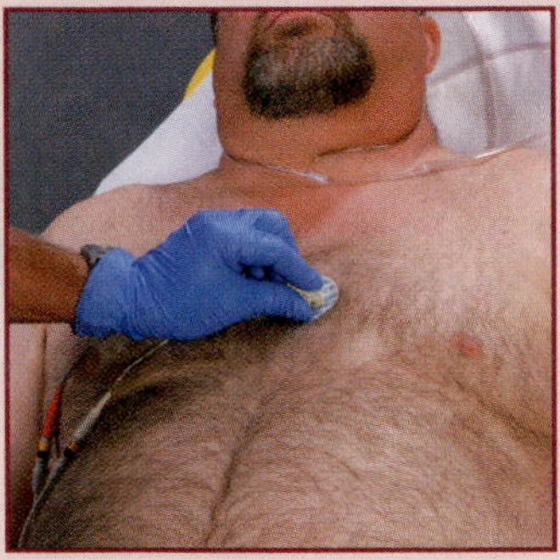

Figure 31.9

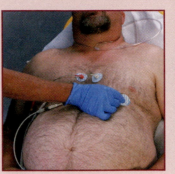

Figure 31.10

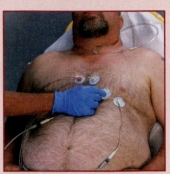

Figure 31.11

7. Place the V_1 lead to the right of the sternum in the 4th intercostal space (Figure 31.8).
8. Place the V_2 lead to the left of the sternum in the 4th intercostal space (Figure 31.9).
9. Place the V_4 lead at the midclavicular line in the 5th intercostal space (Figure 31.10).
10. Place the V_3 lead midway between leads V_2 and V_4 (Figure 31.11).
11. Place the V_5 lead at the anterior axillary line at the same level as V_4 (Figure 31.12).
12. Place the V_6 lead at the midaxillary line at the same level as V_4 and V_5 (Figure 31.13).
13. Ensure that the ECG leads are plugged into the cardiac monitor.

    Rationale: The leads need to be plugged into the cardiac monitor for it to perform the 12-lead ECG.
14. Turn the monitor and the 12-lead ECG function on.

    Rationale: Most cardiac monitors with 12-lead capability have a separate power switch for the 12-lead function.
15. Ask the patient to remain motionless while breathing normally during the 12-lead ECG recording (Figure 31.14).

    Rationale: Patient movement will create artifact, which will lessen the quality of the tracing.
16. Record the 12-lead ECG tracing as described by the unit's manufacturer (Figure 31.15).

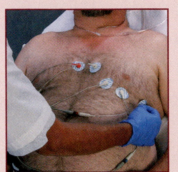

Figure 31.12

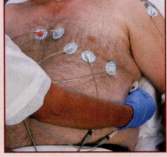

Figure 31.13

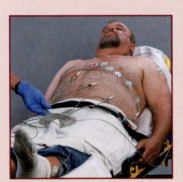

Figure 31.14

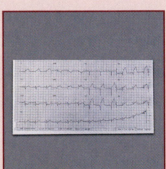

Figure 31.15

Rationale: Different 12-lead ECG units will have different operational methods; it is the responsibility of the paramedic to be familiar with his equipment.

17. Assess the 12-lead ECG tracing to ensure that an adequate tracing has been obtained (Figure 31.16), and then perform rhythm interpretation and explain your findings to the patient (Figure 31.17). If the quality of the ECG tracing is poor, identify and correct the problem and repeat the tracing.

    Rationale: Loose leads, patient movement, or environmental conditions may influence the quality of the ECG tracing. Poor quality 12-lead ECGs should be repeated until an acceptable tracing is obtained to ensure the highest degree of interpretation accuracy.

18. Document any information regarding the 12-lead ECG. Attach any paper tracings that you may have to your patient care report.

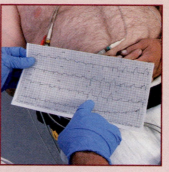

Figure 31.16

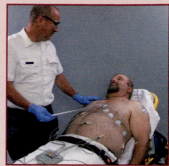

Figure 31.17

ONGOING ASSESSMENT

A patient who requires cardiac monitoring is either serious or unstable and should be reassessed every 5 minutes until his condition stabilizes, at which time reassessment every 15 minutes may be sufficient. Glancing at the cardiac monitor, however, is not acceptable for reassessment. A full set of vitals, including pulse, respirations, and blood pressure, in addition to cardiac rhythm interpretation, should be measured.

Resist the temptation to treat every observable rhythm. Frequently, patients will have a few unusual heart beats that require no treatment at all. If an abnormal rhythm does present on the monitor, confirm the need for treatment with other physical signs such as changes in heart rate, respirations, blood pressure, skin color, or diaphoresis. Additionally, patients experiencing unusual rhythms will often complain of nausea, dizziness, or chest pain or discomfort. Act swiftly with proper treatment when needed, but only if the total patient picture warrants it.

▶ PROBLEM SOLVING

▶ Identification of the Angle of Louis may be difficult on some patients. Remember that the sternum articulates with the clavicle directly superior to the 1st rib. To identify the 1st rib, palpate the clavicle medial to the sternum, then locate the 1st rib immediately inferior to the clavicle.

▶ Proper electrode contact will be difficult in patients with excessive body hair. If you find yourself thinking that a patient may have enough hair to interfere with the 12-lead ECG acquisition, shave the patient!

▶ Diaphoresis can interfere with the adherence of electrodes. The use of tincture of benzoin or commercial "diaphoretic" electrodes can increase electrode adhesiveness, and should be considered immediately rather than trying to replace electrodes or apply benzoin after the application of regular electrodes.

▶ Placing the leads onto the electrode pads is best done before placing the pad on the patient. To apply the lead to the pad, simply snap the button into place on the lead, and then peel off the backing to the pad and stick it on the patient in the correct location. If you place the pad and then try and attach the electrode it can be uncomfortable for the patient. You will usually have to apply a lot of downward pressure, or even pinch the skin to get the button to snap in place.

▶ Normal cardiac monitoring during transport can prove frustrating if you are utilizing limb leads placed on the limbs. After performing the 12-lead ECG, you may want to place the limb leads onto the torso for routine cardiac monitoring. This will significantly reduce artifact produced during normal patient limb movement, and the leads can be quickly reattached to the limbs should a repeat 12-lead ECG be necessary.

▶ The patient should be supine during the 12-lead acquisition. If this is not possible due to dyspnea then document the position of the patient directly on the 12-lead printout so that subsequent 12-leads can be acquired in the same position for comparison purposes.

▶CASE STUDY

You and your paramedic partner have just finished eating breakfast when your ambulance is dispatched to a "dizzy person." You arrive on scene at a private home and are presented with Mrs. Jones, a 38-year-old female in the care of the first-responding engine who is conscious and alert, holding a nonrebreather mask to her face, and obviously embarrassed at the attention she is receiving. While an EMT-Firefighter is taking the patient's vital signs, she describes a brief period of near-syncope and dizziness while she was eating breakfast sitting at the kitchen table. She denies any loss of consciousness, chest pain, difficulty breathing, dizziness, or weakness right now and says that she "is fine" and she does not want to go to the hospital. You note that her skin is cool, pale, and slightly diaphoretic.

You motion for your partner to place the patient on the cardiac monitor, and the husband says that he called 911 because "she became very pale and almost passed out." When you ask, the patient informs you that she has a history of insulin-dependant diabetes and that heart disease runs in her family. The patient's vital signs are a pulse of 90, respiratory rate of 14, blood pressure of 118/68, and a SaO_2 of 100 percent on 15 lpm via the nonrebreather mask. The cardiac monitor shows a normal sinus rhythm, and a fingerstick reveals a blood glucose of 124 mg/dL. The patient states that she does not want to go to the hospital, but you explain to her that her description of the event and her past medical and family history concern you and you would like to perform a 12-lead ECG. She agrees, saying "When it comes back fine I can go to work!"

You attach the 12-lead cables to the monitor, place the diaphoretic electrodes on the lead cables, and proceed to identify the 4th intercostal space. You find the Angle of Louis, identify the 1st rib and intercostal space, then count down to the 4th intercostal space. You place V_1 in the 4th intercostal space just to the right of the sternum, V_2 in the 4th intercostal space just to the left of the sternum, V_4 in the 5th intercostal space at the midclavicular line, and V_3 between V_2 and V_4. You then identify the anterior axillary and midaxillary lines and place V_5 and V_6 at the same level of V_4. You note that your partner has moved the limb leads from the patient's torso to her limbs, turned the 12-lead function of the cardiac monitor on, instructed the patient to lie motionless during the procedure, and recorded a tracing. Upon reviewing the printout, you are immediately able to identify 4 mm of ST segment elevation in leads V_3–V_5. "Mrs. Jones," you say, "I think that I know why you were dizzy." ■

GLOSSARY

Abrasions scratches or scrapes.

Absolute refractory period stage of cell activity in which the cardiac cell cannot spontaneously depolarize.

Absorption passage of a substance through skin or mucous membranes upon contact.

Acetone wipe a cleaning agent containing a chemical solvent.

Activated charcoal a powder, usually premixed with water, that will absorb some poisons and will prevent them from being absorbed by the body.

Adult respiratory distress syndrome (ARDS) respiratory insufficiency marked by progressive hypoxemia, due to severe inflammatory damage.

Agonal respiration a gasping-type respiration that has no pattern and occurs very infrequently; a sign of impending cardiac or respiratory arrest. *Also called* agonal breathing.

Air embolism an air bubble that enters the bloodstream and obstructs a blood vessel.

Airborne particles particles transported by air.

Alkali a strong base, especially the metallic hydroxides. Alkalis combine with acids to form salts, combine with fatty acids to form soap, neutralize acids, and turn litmus paper blue.

Altered level of consciousness situation where a patient is in a questionable mental state, ranging from sleep to a coma.

Altered mental status a condition in which the patient displays a change in his normal mental state ranging from disorientation to complete unresponsiveness.

Alveoli microscopic air sacs in the lungs where most oxygen and carbon dioxide gas exchanges take place.

Ambulatory able to walk; not confined to bed.

Amniotic sac the "bag of waters" that surrounds the developing fetus.

Amputation the surgical removal or traumatic severing of a body part, usually an extremity.

Anaphylaxis an unusual or exaggerated allergic reaction to a foreign protein or other substance.

Anatomical disturbances body-related abnormalities.

Anemia when blood lacks red blood cells, hemoglobin, or total volume.

Angina pain in the chest, occurring when blood supply to the heart is reduced and a portion of the heart muscle is not receiving enough oxygen.

Angioedema a condition marked by the development of edematous areas of skin, mucous membranes, or internal organs.

Angle of the jaw the angle formed by the junction of the posterior edge of the ramus of the mandible and the lower surface of the body of the mandible.

Ankle hitch traction device that slides over and stabilizes the ankle.

Antecubital fossa triangular area lying anterior to and below the elbow, bounded medially by the pronator teres and laterally by the brachioradialis muscles.

Anterior-axillary line a vertical skin fold along the anterior axillary fold; crease of the underarm.

Antidote substance that will neutralize the poison or its effects.

Aphagia inability to swallow.

Apical pulse the pulse felt or heard over the lower part of the heart.

Apnea absence of breathing.

Areflexic areflexia: absence of reflexes.

Artifact electrical activity displayed on graph paper that is superimposed on cardiac tracings, interfering with interpretation of the rhythm. *Also called* interference.

Artificial ventilation forcing air or oxygen into the lungs when a patient has stopped breathing or has inadequate breathing. *Also called* positive-pressure ventilation.

Aseptic technique a method used in surgery to prevent contamination of the wound and operative site. All instruments used are sterilized, and physicians and nurses wear caps, masks, shoe coverings, sterile gowns, and gloves.

Aspiration breathing a foreign substance into the lungs.

Asystole the absence of any cardiac electrical activity.

Atrial fibrillation the cardiac arrhythmia in which the atria are controlled by numerous irritable foci, thereby causing ineffectual, chaotic atrial activity and irregular ventricular response.

Auscultate Listen. A stethoscope is used to auscultate for characteristic body sounds.

Automated external defibrillator (AED) a device that can analyze the electrical activity or rhythm of a patient's heart and deliver an electrical shock (defibrillation) if appropriate.

Avulsion the tearing away or tearing off of a piece or flap of skin or other soft tissue. This term also may be used for an eye pulled from its socket or a tooth dislodged from its socket.

Bag-valve-mask ventilation artificial ventilation to a patient via squeezing a handheld device with a face mask and self-refilling bag. Can deliver air from the atmosphere or oxygen from a supplemental oxygen supply system.

Bandage any material used to hold a dressing in place.

Barotrauma injury caused by pressure within an enclosed space.

Baseline mental status a control measurement used for comparisons when determining altered mental states.

Baseline vital signs the first set of vital signs measurements to which subsequent measurements can be compared.

Bifurcation a separation into two branches; the point of forking.

Biphasic a single EKG wave that has two deflections, one upright and the other inverted.

Biphasic energy levels defibrillation shocks that are first administered in one direction, and then another.

Body mechanics the proper use of the body to facilitate lifting and moving and prevent injury.

Bone marrow the soft tissue in the marrow cavities of long bones (yellow marrow) and in the spaces between trabeculae of spongy bone in the sternum and other flat and irregular bones.

Brachial pulse the pulse felt in the upper arm; the pulse checked during infant CPR.

Bradycardia a heart rate that is less than 60 beats per minute.

Bronchioles smaller branches of the bronchi that continue to branch and get smaller, eventually leading into alveolar sacs.

Bronchodilator therapy use of a medicine to enlarge constricted bronchial tubes, making breathing easier.

Bronchodilators drugs that relax the smooth muscle of the bronchi and bronchioles and reverse bronchoconstriction.

Broselow® tape a measuring tape for infants that provides important information regarding airway equipment and medication doses based on the patient's length.

BSI equipment body substance isolation equipment, consisting of gloves, masks, and goggles, used to prevent the spread of disease through pathogens.

BSI precautions steps taken to prevent the spread of disease through blood-borne or air-borne pathogens.

Burns tissue injury resulting from excessive exposure to thermal, chemical, electrical, or radioactive agents.

Cannula hollow needle used to puncture a vein.

Cannulate to introduce a cannula through a passageway.

Capnography a recording or display of the measurement of exhaled carbon dioxide concentrations.

Capnometry the measurement of the concentration of carbon dioxide in the exhaled breath of a critically ill person.

Carbon monoxide poisoning toxicity that results from inhalation of small amounts of carbon monoxide over a long period or from large amounts inhaled for a short time.

Cardioversion a maneuver used to convert various tachyarrhythmias to more viable rhythms; consists of application of electrical countershock (DC current) to the chest wall; the electrical discharge is usually synchronized to fall on the R wave, thus avoiding the relative refractory period.

Carina the fork at the lower end of the trachea where the two mainstem bronchi branch.

Carotid pulse the pulse felt along the large carotid artery on either side of the neck.

Catheter a tube passed through the body for evacuating fluids or injecting them into body cavities.

Caustic solutions an agent that burns or dissolves organic tissue through chemical action.

Caustic substance an agent, particularly an alkali, that destroys living tissue.

Cervical collar device placed around the neck to stabilize the spinal column in the event of a suspected injury.

Chief complaint in emergency medicine, the reason EMS was called, usually in the patient's own words.

Childbirth the physiological process by which the fetus is expelled from the uterus into the vagina and then to the outside of the body. *Also called* labor.

Chronic pulmonary disease umbrella term used to describe pulmonary diseases such as emphysema or chronic bronchitis.

Circumferential encircling a body area (e.g., arm, leg, or chest).

Clavicle the collarbone.

Colormetric device a device that changes color in the presence of CO_2.

Constipation a decrease in a person's normal frequency of defecation accompanied by difficult or incomplete passage of stool and/or passage of excessively hard, dry stool.

Continuous positive airway pressure (CPAP) a method by which positive airway pressure is maintained throughout the respiratory cycle; can be administered through a face mask, nasal mask, or an endotracheal tube.

Contraction a shortening or tightening, as of a muscle; a shrinking or reduction in size.

Contusions bruises; in brain injuries, a bruised brain caused when the force of a blow to the head is great enough to rupture blood vessels.

Cravat a band or scarf worn around the neck.

Crepitation the grating sound or feeling of broken bones rubbing together. *Also called* crepitus.

Crepitus the sound or feel of broken fragments of bone grinding against each other.

Cricoid cartilage the ring-shaped structure that circles the trachea at the lower end of the larynx.

Cricoid pressure pressure applied to the cricoid cartilage to compress the esophagus. *Also called* Sellick's maneuver.

Cross-finger technique a technique in which the thumb and index finger are crossed, with the thumb on the lower incisors and the index finger on the

upper incisors. The fingers are moved in a snapping or scissor motion to open the mouth.

Crowning when part of the baby is visible through the vaginal opening.

Cyanide a rapid-acting agent that disrupts the ability of the cell to use oxygen, leading to severe cellular hypoxia and eventual death.

Cyanosis a blue or gray color resulting from lack of oxygen in the body.

D_5W a carbohydrate solution that uses glucose (sugar) as the solute dissolved in sterile water. Five percent dextrose in water is packed as an isotonic solution but becomes hypotonic once in the body because the glucose (solute) dissolved in sterile water is metabolized by the body's cells.

Debridement the removal of foreign material and dead or damaged tissue, especially in a wound.

Defibrillation electrical shock or current delivered to the heart through the patient's chest wall to help the heart restore a normal rhythm.

Deformity alteration in the natural form of a part or organ; distortion of any part or general disfigurement of the body. It may be acquired or congenital. If present after injury, deformity usually implies the presence of fracture, dislocation, or both. It may be due to extensive swelling, extravasation of blood, or rupture of muscles.

Diabetes *also called* "sugar diabetes," the condition brought about by decreased insulin production or the inability of the body cells to use insulin properly. The person with this condition is a diabetic.

Diaphoresis profuse sweating.

Diastolic blood pressure the pressure remaining in the arteries when the left ventricle of the heart is relaxed and refilling.

Dislocation the disruption or "coming apart" of a joint.

Distal farther away from the torso. *Opposite of* proximal.

Do not resuscitate (DNR) order a legal document, usually signed by the patient and his or her physician, which states that the patient has a terminal illness and does not wish to prolong life through resuscitative efforts.

Dorsalis pedal pulse pulse taken at the artery supplying blood to the foot, lateral to the large tendon of the big toe.

Dressing any material (preferably sterile) used to cover a wound that will help control bleeding and help prevent additional contamination.

Dysphagia inability to swallow or difficulty swallowing.

Dysphonia difficulty in speaking; hoarseness.

Dysrhythmia a disturbance in heart rate and rhythm.

Ectopic focus nonpacemaker heart cell that automatically depolarizes causing irregular heart beats or heart rhythms; *pl.* ectopic foci.

Edema swelling resulting from buildup of fluid in the tissues.

Electrode metal wire attached to the patient's body for the purpose of conveying electrical impulses to a machine for recording or displaying.

Endotracheal (ET) intubation placement of a tube down the trachea to facilitate airflow into the lungs and aid in breathing.

Endotracheal (ET) tube a tube designed to be inserted into the trachea. Oxygen, medication, or a suction catheter can be directed into the trachea through an endotracheal tube.

Epiglottis a leaf-shaped structure that prevents food and foreign matter from entering the trachea.

Epinephrine a natural hormone that, when used as a medication, constricts blood vessels to improve blood pressure, reduces leakage from blood vessels, and relaxes smooth muscle in the bronchioles.

Epinephrine auto-injector a syringe with a spring-loaded needle that administers epinephrine to patients who are susceptible to severe allergic reactions.

Esophageal Intubation Detector (EID) a device used to verify endotracheal tube placement using negative pressure; also Esophageal Detector Device.

Esophageal Tracheal Combitube® (ETC) a double lumen airway where the two lumens are separated by a partition wall; used on unconscious patients over five feet tall.

Esophagus the tube that leads from the pharynx to the stomach.

Evisceration an intestine or other internal organ protruding through a wound in the abdomen.

Exsanguination massive bleeding.

Extravasation the escape of fluid from its physiologic contained space (e.g., blood into the surrounding tissue).

Extremity the portions of the skeleton that include the clavicles, scapulae, arms, wrists, and hands (upper extremities) and the pelvis, thighs, legs, ankles, and feet (lower extremities).

Extubation the removal of a tube.

Eye protection personal protective equipment such as goggles used to prevent illness or injury from affecting the eyes.

Femoral pulse pulse found in the major artery supplying the leg; can be found in the crease between the abdomen and groin.

Field impression evaluation of the environment to ascertain if a patient is in further danger because of location.

Flowmeter a valve that indicates the flow of oxygen in liters per minute.

Flutter valve a catheter device that prevents air from flowing into the chest cavity during inspiration, while allowing for the venting off of re-accumulating pressure.

Focused history the step of patient assessment that follows the initial assessment and includes the patient history, physical exam, and vital signs.

Fontanelle the "soft spot" on the top of an infant's head where the plates of the skull have not yet formed together.

Formable splint splints that can be molded to different angles, and therefore allow considerable movement.

Fracture any break in a bone.

French (unit of measure) a European term for a size of tubing equivalent to about .013 thousandths of an inch; the larger the number, the larger the catheter.

Gag reflex vomiting or retching that results when something is placed in the back of the pharynx.

Gastric distension inflation of the stomach.

Gastric extension enlargement of the stomach.

General impression impression of the patient's condition that is formed on first approaching the patient, based on the patient's environment, chief complaint, and appearance.

Glottic opening the opening to the trachea.

Gloves a protective covering for the hand. In medical care, the glove is made of a flexible, impervious material that permits full movement of the fingers. Gloves are used to protect both the operative site from contamination with organisms from the health care worker and the health care worker from contamination with pathogens from the patient.

Glucagon substance that increases the blood glucose level.

Glucose monitoring process whereby people with diabetes determine the level of glucose in the blood, which dictates how much insulin should be taken.

Gown a coverall worn in an operating room.

Handheld nebulizer portable device capable of emitting a fine spray.

HARE traction splint splint used for femur fractures that helps immobilize the leg during transport.

Head tilt-chin lift maneuver a means of correcting blockage of the airway by the tongue by tilting the head back and lifting the chin. Used when no trauma, or injury, is suspected. *See also* jaw-thrust maneuver.

Heart blocks interference with the normal transmission of electrical impulses through the conducting system of the heart.

Hematoma collection of blood beneath the skin or trapped within a body compartment.

Hemodynamically unstable situation where abnormalities exist in the circulation of the blood.

Hemoglobin a complex protein molecule found on the surface of the red blood cell that is responsible for carrying a majority of oxygen in the blood.

Hemorrhage bleeding, especially severe bleeding.

Heparin a parenteral anticoagulant drug used in the prevention and treatment of thrombosis and embolism.

High-priority conditions situations that require immediate attention; include unresponsive, difficult breathing, shock, uncontrolled bleeding, severe pain, or complicated childbirth.

Humerus the bone of the upper arm, between the shoulder and the elbow.

Hydrocarbon a compound made up primarily of hydrogen and carbon.

Hydrochloric acid an aqueous solution of hydrogen chloride that is a strong corrosive irritating acid, is normally present in dilute form in gastric juice, and is widely used in industry and in the laboratory.

Hypercapnia an increased amount of carbon dioxide in the blood.

Hypercarbia an increased amount of carbon dioxide in the blood.

Hyperextension extreme or abnormal extension.

Hypersensitivity an exaggerated and harmful immune response.

Hyperventilate to provide ventilations at a higher rate than normal.

Hyperventilation increased minute volume ventilation, which results in a lowered carbon dioxide level. It is a frequent finding in many disease processes such as asthma, metabolic acidosis, pulmonary embolism, and pulmonary edema, and also in anxiety-induced states.

Hypocarbia a decreased amount of carbon dioxide in the blood.

Hypodermic needle hollow metal tube used with the syringe to administer medications.

Hypoglycemia low blood sugar.

Hypoperfusion shock; inadequate perfusion of the cells and tissues of the body caused by insufficient flow of blood through the capillaries. *See also* perfusion.

Hypotension a deficiency in tone or tension; a decrease of the systolic and diastolic blood pressure to below normal. This occurs, for example, in shock, hemorrhage, dehydration, sepsis, Addison's disease, and in many other diseases and conditions.

Hypoventilation reduced rate and depth of breathing that causes an increase in carbon dioxide.

Hypovolemic shock shock resulting from blood or fluid loss.

Hypoxemia decreased blood oxygen level.

Hypoxia an insufficiency of oxygen in the body's tissues.

Immobilization the making of a part or limb immovable.

Impaled object an object embedded in an injury to the body.

Index of suspicion awareness that there may be injuries.

Infection control plan a written policy required of all agencies that details the steps to follow in the event of exposure to infectious substances.

Infectious diseases illnesses spread by contact with patients carrying viruses or bacteria; minimized through the use of personal protective equipment.

Inferior away from the head; usually compared with another structure that is closer to the head (e.g., the lips are inferior to the nose). *Opposite of* superior.

Infiltrate to pass into or through a substance or a space.

Initial assessment the first element in assessment of a patient; steps taken for the purpose of discovering and dealing with any life-threatening problems. The six parts of initial assessment are: forming a general impression, assessing mental status, assessing airway, assessing breathing, assessing circulation, and determining the priority of the patient for treatment and transport to the hospital.

In-line stabilization bringing the patient's head into a neutral position in which the nose is lined up with the navel and holding it there manually.

Inspection visual examination of the external surface of the body as well as of its movements and posture.

Intercostal space between the ribs.

Intramuscular within the muscle.

Intramuscular injection (IM) injection into a muscle.

Intravenous within or into a vein.

Intubation insertion of a tube.

Ischial strap device used for support of the ischium, or posterior portion of the pelvis.

Ischium the lower, posterior portions of the pelvis.

Jaundiced skin yellowness of the skin.

Jaw-thrust maneuver a means of correcting blockage of the airway by moving the jaw forward without tilting the head or neck. Used when trauma, or injury, is suspected to open the airway without causing further injury to the spinal cord in the neck. *See also* head tilt-chin lift maneuver.

Kendrick extrication device (KED) a vest-type immobilizer designed to limit movement of the cervical and thoracic spine in seated patients with suspected spinal cord injuries.

Kinematics the branch of biomechanics concerned with description of the movements of segments of the body without regard to the forces that caused the movement to occur.

Kling soft, flexible roller-gauze used in dressing and bandaging.

Lacerations cuts; in brain injuries, a cut to the brain.

Laryngectomy a surgical procedure in which a patient's larynx is removed. A stoma is created for the patient to breathe through.

Laryngoscope an illuminating instrument that is inserted into the pharynx to permit visualization of the pharynx and larynx.

Laryngoscopy the procedure of using a laryngoscope to lift the epiglottis to visualize the vocal cords and glottic opening.

Laryngospasm spasm of the laryngeal muscles.

Lateral position to the side; away from the midline of the body.

Lead an electrocardiographic view of the heart, gained by recording the electrical activity between two or more electrodes.

Level of consciousness varying stages of patient awareness.

Level of distress evaluation of the amount of pain or distress within the patient.

Life threats situation in which a patient is in need of immediate action for survival.

Lifting devices equipment used to elevate patients from the ground.

Low-flow oxygen method of delivering oxygen to a patient through nasal cannulas inserted in the nose.

Lumen the tunnel through a tube.

Magill forceps angulated forceps used during direct laryngoscopy to remove a foreign body from an obstructed airway.

Mandible the lower jaw bone.

Manual defibrillation older defibrillation method where an operator reviews a patient's heart rhythm, decides it is shockable, lubricates two paddles, and delivers a shock to the patient's chest.

Manual traction the process of applying tension to straighten and realign a fractured limb before splinting. *Also called* tension.

Mask a covering for the face that serves as a protective barrier.

MAST medical anti-shock trousers.

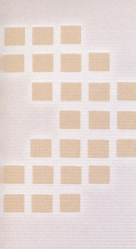

Mechanism of injury (MOI) a force or forces that may have caused injury.

Metered-dose inhaler (MDI) device consisting of a plastic container and a canister of medication that is used to inhale an aerosolized medication.

Midaxillary line an imaginary line that divides the body into anterior and posterior planes; the imaginary line from the middle of the armpit to the ankle.

Midclavicular line the line through the center of each clavicle.

Midshaft femur thick portion of the lower leg bone.

Monophasic energy levels sending energy in one direction.

Mucous plugs clots of mucus built up in the lungs, which can block the airway if coughed up.

Myocardial infarction the loss of living heart muscle as a result of coronary artery occlusion.

Nares the nostrils.

Nasal cannula a device that delivers low concentrations of oxygen through two prongs that rest in the patient's nostrils.

Nasogastric (NG) tube a tube designed to be passed through the nose, nasopharynx, and esophagus. It is used to relieve distension of the stomach in an infant or child patient.

Nasopharyngeal airway (NPA) a flexible breathing tube inserted through the patient's nose into the pharynx to help maintain an open airway.

Nasopharynx the airway directly posterior to the nose.

Nature of the illness what is medically wrong with a patient.

Nebulizer chamber an apparatus for producing a fine spray or mist. This may be done by rapidly passing air through a liquid or by vibrating a liquid at a high frequency so that the particles produced are extremely small.

Necrosis cell death; a pathological cell change.

Needle decompression surgical puncture of the chest wall for removal or instillation of fluids.

Neutral alignment the position of bones in anatomical position, without excessive extension, flexion, or rotation.

Neutrally aligned position the position of bones in anatomical position, without excessive extension, flexion, or rotation.

Nitroglycerin a drug that helps to dilate the coronary vessels that supply the heart muscle with blood.

Nitroglycerin patch adhesive-backed material that administers nitroglycerin through the skin (dermal administration) several times a day.

Nonmetallic surface area that does not contain the chemical properties of a metal.

Nonrebreather mask a face mask and reservoir bag device that delivers high concentrations of oxygen. The patient's exhaled air escapes through a valve and is not rebreathed.

Nonurgent moves patient moves made when no immediate threat to life exists.

Normal saline solution an isotonic crystalloid solution that contains sodium chloride (salt) as the solute, dissolved in sterile water (solvent). The specific concentration for normal saline solution is 0.9 percent.

Nostril one of the external apertures of the nose.

Occiput the back part of the skull.

Occlusive dressing any dressing that forms an airtight seal.

One-way valve valve that allows movement in only one direction, such as the valve that prevents blood from being forced back up the atrium.

Ongoing assessment a procedure for detecting changes in a patient's condition. It involves four steps: repeating the initial assessment, repeating and recording vital signs, repeating the focused assessment, and checking interventions.

Open wounds an injury in which the skin is interrupted, exposing the tissue beneath.

Oral glucose a form of glucose (a kind of sugar) given by mouth to treat an awake patient (who is able to swallow) with an altered mental status and a history of diabetes.

Orbits the bony structures around the eyes; the eye sockets.

Organic solvents naturally occurring compound used to dissolve or disperse other substances.

Oropharyngeal airway (OPA) a curved device inserted through the patient's mouth into the pharynx to help maintain an open airway.

Oxygen regulator a device connected to an oxygen cylinder that reduces pressure to a safe level for the patient to intake.

Oxygen saturation percentage the ratio of the amount of oxygen present in the blood to the amount that could be carried, expressed as a percentage.

Oxygenation the process by which the blood and the cells become saturated with oxygen.

Oxygen saturation the saturation of arterial blood with oxygen as measured by pulse oximetry; expressed as a percentage.

Oxytocin a pituitary hormone that stimulates the uterus to contract, thus inducing parturition. It also acts on the mammary gland to stimulate the release of milk.

Pacemaker in cardiology, a specialized cell or group of cells that automatically regenerates impulses that spread to other regions of the heart. The normal cardiac pacemaker is the sinoatrial node, a group of cells in the right atrium near the entrance of the superior vena cava. A generally accepted term for artificial cardiac pacemaker.

Painful stimulus an agent that causes extreme discomfort for the patient.

Palpated blood pressure procedure where the radial or brachial pulse is felt with the fingertips to determine blood pressure; not as accurate as auscultated blood pressure, but is sometimes used when there is too much noise for a stethoscope to be effective.

Palpation touching or feeling. A pulse or blood pressure may be palpated with the fingertips.

Paradoxical motion movement of a part of the chest in the opposite direction to the rest of the chest during respiration.

Parietal pleura the outermost pleural layer that adheres to the chest wall.

Paroxysmal sudden onset and cessation; often used to describe atrial tachycardia if it is characterized by abrupt onset and termination.

PASG pneumatic anti-shock garment.

Past medical history record of previous medical issues and procedures that may be used to help the physician with diagnosis or treatment.

Pathogens the organisms that cause infection, such as viruses and bacteria.

Penetrations injuries caused by an object that passes through the skin or other body tissues.

Perfusion the supply of oxygen to and removal of wastes from the cells and tissues of the body as a result of the flow of blood through the capillaries. *See also* hypoperfusion.

Periorbital ecchymosis black and blue discoloration surrounding the socket of the eye.

Pharyngeal relating to or located or produced in the region of the pharynx.

Pharynx the area directly posterior to the mouth and nose. It is made up of the oropharynx and the nasopharynx.

Pin-index safety system a means by which anesthesiologists prevent misconnection to the wrong yoke.

Placenta the organ of pregnancy where exchange of oxygen, foods, and wastes occurs between a mother and fetus.

Pleural space small space between the visceral and parietal pleura that is at negative pressure and filled with serous fluid.

Pneumonia infection of the lungs, usually from a bacterium or virus.

Pneumothorax air in the chest cavity, outside the lungs.

Pocket mask a device, usually with a one-way valve, to aid in artificial ventilation. A rescuer breathes through the valve when the mask is placed over the patient's face. Also acts as a barrier to prevent contact with a patient's breath or body fluids. Can be used with supplemental oxygen when fitted with an oxygen inlet.

Positional asphyxia death of a person due to a body position that restricts breathing for a prolonged period of time.

Posterior the back of the body or body part. *Opposite of* anterior.

Power grip gripping with as much hand surface as possible in contact with the object being lifted, all fingers bent at the same angle, hands at least 10 inches apart.

Power lift a lift from a squatting position with weight to be lifted close to the body, feet apart and flat on the ground, body weight on or just behind balls of feet, back locked in. The upper body is raised before the hips. *Also called* the squat-lift position.

Preoxygenation breathing of 100 percent oxygen via a face mask by the fully conscious patient.

Presenting problem the illness or injury for which the patient is seeking medical attention.

Proximal closer to the torso. *Opposite of* distal.

Pulse the rhythmic beats felt as the heart pumps blood through the arteries.

Pulse oximeter an electronic device for determining the amount of oxygen carried in the blood, and the oxygen saturation or SpO_2.

Pulseless electrical activity (PEA) the absence of a palpable pulse and myocardial muscle activity with the presence of organized electrical activity on the cardiac monitor.

Punctures open wounds that tear through the skin and destroy underlying tissues. A *penetrating puncture wound* can be shallow or deep. A *perforating puncture wound* has both an entrance and an exit wound.

R wave the first upright deflection following the P wave, or the first positive wave of the QRS complex.

Radial pulse the pulse felt at the wrist.

Rales crackles.

Rapid extrication a technique using manual stabilization rather than application of an immobilization device for the purpose of speeding extrication when the time saved will make the difference between life and death.

Rapid trauma assessment a rapid assessment of the head, neck, chest, abdomen, pelvis, extremities, and posterior of the body to detect signs and symptoms of injury.

Reasonable force the minimum amount of force required to keep a patient from injuring himself or others.

Reduce to restore to usual relationship, as the ends of a fractured bone. To weaken, as a solution. To diminish, as bulk or weight.

Reservoir bag a container that can hold air in a breathing apparatus.

Respiration breathing.

Rigid splint splint made of cardboard, wood, or pneumatic devices that requires the limb to be moved to the anatomical position, which provides the greatest support.

Ringer's lactate an isotonic crystalloid solution containing the solutes sodium chloride, potassium chloride, calcium chloride, and sodium lactate, dissolved in sterile water (solvent).

Roller gauze a strip of muslin or other cloth rolled up in cylinder form for surgical use. A roller bandage.

Sager traction splint unipolar traction splint that continuously shows the amount of traction being applied.

Saline containing or pertaining to salt.

Scapula the shoulder blade.

Sellick's maneuver pressure applied to the cricoid cartilage to compress the esophagus. *Also called* cricoid pressure.

Septum a wall dividing two cavities.

Serial vital signs an ongoing monitoring of body systems.

Severe allergic reaction an allergic reaction where the patient has either respiratory distress or indications of shock.

Shock management treatment procedures to assist a patient in shock; includes maintaining an open airway, providing oxygen, elevating the legs, and protecting the patient from heat loss.

Shoulder girdle the two scapulae and two clavicles attaching the bones of the upper extremities to the axial skeleton.

Sling and swathe a support for an injured upper extremity.

Soft restraints items such as leather cuffs and belts that can be used to hold patients while minimizing the chance for soft-tissue injury.

Soft-tip suction catheter a dilatation and curettage device designed to minimize trauma under certain conditions.

Sphygmomanometer the cuff and gauge used to measure blood pressure.

Splint any device used to immobilize a body part.

Spontaneous respirations automatic process of bringing oxygen into the body and distributing it throughout the body.

Standing takedown process of carefully but rapidly taking a standing patient down to the supine position to prevent spinal injury.

Stoma a permanent surgical opening in the neck through which the patient breathes.

Stridor a harsh, high-pitched sound heard on inspiration that indicates swelling of the larynx.

Stylette a long, thin, flexible metal probe.

Subcutaneous beneath the skin.

Subcutaneous injection (SQ) injection beneath the skin.

Suction use of a vacuum device to remove blood, vomitus, and other secretions or foreign materials from the airway.

Supine position lying on the back *Opposite of* prone.

Supplemental oxygen additional oxygen that is forced into a patient's lungs during periods of inadequate or absent breathing; accomplished through oxygen cylinders, pressure regulators, and a delivery device.

Supraventricular tachycardia term used to describe a rapid arrhythmia that is regular, has no visible P waves, and has a rate range common to other arrhythmias, thereby making more accurate identification impossible; loosely used to refer to any tachycardia that originated above the ventricles.

Sutures thread, wire, or other material used to stitch parts of the body together. The seam or line of union formed by surgical stitches.

Swelling an abnormal transient enlargement, especially one appearing on the surface of the body. Ice applied to the area helps to limit swelling.

Symptomatic of the nature of or concerning a symptom.

Synchronous occurring simultaneously.

Systolic blood pressure the pressure created when the heart contracts and forces blood out into the arteries.

Tachycardia a rapid heart rate; any pulse rate above 100 beats per minute.

Tachypnea a breathing rate that is faster than the normal rate.

Tenderness pain in response to palpation.

Tension pneumothorax a condition in which the buildup of air and pressure in the thoracic cavity of the injured lung is so severe that it begins to shift to the uninjured side, resulting in compression of the heart, large vessels, and the uninjured lung.

Thermoregulatory pertaining to the regulation of temperature, especially body temperature.

Thyroid cartilage the bulky, shield-like structure, commonly known as the Adams's apple, that forms the anterior surface of the larynx.

Tidal volume the volume of air breathed in and out during one respiration.

Tissue necrosis tissue death.

Tongue blade a thin instrument rounded at the ends used to depress the tongue to inspect the mouth and throat; *also called* a tongue depressor.

Torsades de Pointes a rapid, unstable form of ventricular tachycardia in which the QRS complexes appear to twist, or shift, electrical orientation around an isoelectric line of the electrocardiogram.

Traction splint a splint that applies constant pull along the length of a lower extremity to help stabilize the fractured bone and to reduce muscle spasm in the limb. Traction splints are used primarily on femoral shaft fractures.

Trendelenburg positioning a position in which the patient's feet and legs are higher than the head. *Also called* shock position.

Trimester a three-month period.

Tripod positioning a position in which the patient sits upright, leans slightly forward, and supports the body with the arms in front and elbows locked. This is a common position found in respiratory distress.

Trismus tonic contraction of the muscles of mastication; lockjaw.

Trocar a sharply pointed surgical instrument contained in a cannula; used for aspiration or removal of fluids from cavities.

T-tube tube inserted into the thoracic cavity.

Umbilical cord the fetal structure containing the blood vessels that carry blood to and from the placenta.

Unresponsive patient person who does not react to a stimulus or treatment.

Unresponsiveness a condition of not reacting to a stimulus or treatment.

Upper airway the portion of the respiratory system that extends from the nose and mouth to the larynx.

Urgent moves patient moves made because there is an immediate threat to life due to the patient's condition and the patient must be moved quickly for transport.

Uvula the free edge of the soft palate that hangs at the back of the throat above the root of the tongue; it is made of muscle, connective tissue, and mucous membrane.

Vallecula depression between the epiglottis and the base of the tongue.

Vascular compromise trauma or disruption of the circulatory system.

Vasodilator a nerve or drug that dilates blood vessels.

Vegetative state a state of severe mental impairment where only involuntary functions are sustained.

Venipuncture puncture of a vein, typically to obtain a specimen of blood.

Ventilation the mechanical process that moves air into and out of the lungs.

Ventricular fibrillation (VF) a condition in which the heart's electrical impulses are disorganized, preventing the heart muscle from contracting normally.

Ventricular tachycardia (VT) a condition in which the heartbeat is quite rapid; if rapid enough, ventricular tachycardia will not allow the heart's chambers to fill with enough blood between beats to produce blood flow sufficient to meet the body's needs.

Visceral pleura innermost layer of the pleura that covers the lung.

Water-soluble lubricant material used to reduce friction that dissolves in water.

Wheezing the production of whistling sounds during difficult breathing such as occurs in asthma, coryza, croup, and other respiratory disorders.

Xiphoid process the inferior portion of the sternum.

INDEX

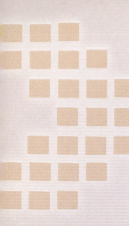

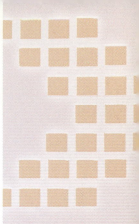